Key Concepts in Health Care Policy and Planning

An introductory text

Colin Palfrey

First published 2000 by
MACMILLAN PRESS LTD
Houndmills, Basingstoke, Hampshire RG21 6XS
and London
Companies and representatives
throughout the world

ISBN 0–333–77740–9

A catalogue record for this book is available
from the British Library.

This book is printed on paper suitable for recycling and
made from fully managed and sustained forest sources.

10 9 8 7 6 5 4 3 2 1
09 08 07 06 05 04 03 02 01 00

Editing and origination by
Aardvark Editorial, Mendham, Suffolk

Printed and bound in Great Britain by
Creative Print & Design (Wales), Ebbw Vale

Key Concepts in Health Care Policy and Planning

Also by Colin Palfrey:

With Nancy Harding
The Social Construction of Dementia
Jessica Kingsley, London, 1997

With Ceri Phillips and Paul Thomas
Evaluating Health and Social Care
Macmillan, Basingstoke, 1994

With Ceri Phillips, Paul Thomas and David Edwards
Policy Evaluation in the Public Sector
Avebury, Aldershot, 1992

To Siân-Elin, Lisa, Dafydd, Gareth and Catrin

Contents

Acknowledgements

I am grateful to a number of people who have, in different ways, contributed to the writing of this book: to the students at the University College of Wales, Swansea and to so many mature students in Hong Kong, Malaysia, Singapore, Saudi Arabia and Mauritius who have expanded my knowledge of different health care systems; to Richenda Milton-Thompson of Macmillan, whose prompt attention and keen interest has been a stimulus to completing the book; to the two reviewers of the original manuscript for their entirely constructive and helpful observations; and particularly to all the authors cited in this volume, without whose scholarship the book could never have been written.

Every effort has been made to trace all the copyright holders but if any have been inadvertently overlooked the publishers will be pleased to make the necessary arrangements at the first opportunity.

Introduction

Aims of the book

This introductory text has developed from extended lecture notes provided for students at home and abroad enrolled on the MSc in Health Care Management course within the Institute of Health Care Studies at the University of Wales, Swansea. The focus is on explaining and illustrating the key concepts that feature prominently in discussions at both national and international level about the kinds of health care system that need to be developed and sustained.

In my travels overseas in order to present the material contained in this book, I have been privileged to meet, as mature students and as colleagues, a wide range of professionals – physicians, nurses, managers, therapists and technicians – working within various health care sectors and services in a number of countries. All of us share similar concerns about the accessibility and quality of services designed to enhance people's quality of life.

Although the main reference point in this book is the British National Health Service (NHS), there is no claim being asserted here that the NHS constitutes a model for any other country to copy or adopt. In many of the countries that I visit as a lecturer, there has been a legacy of the British approach to organising health care services, but, for good reasons, the model has been adapted, modified or rejected. My particular interest has been to study other health care systems in order to understand why and how they are structured in the way they are, and to explore areas of interest and concern that are common to many different health care contexts.

The main aims of the book are these: to offer a conceptual framework to use as a means of analysing the policy process and of appreciating the complexities of health care planning, and to communicate the key concepts that inform this framework in a form that is accessible to busy people, many of whom are studying part time and whose first language is not English. These are modest aims, but in saying this, I am reminded of the politician who remarked about a late-departed adversary: 'He was a modest man and he had much to be modest about'!

I hope that this introductory text will prove useful to students who intend to work or who are already working in health and health care services in the UK and other countries, to students enrolled on courses that relate to public and social policy, and to anyone with an interest in a structured approach to studying an aspect of society that is likely to remain a major challenge to governments throughout the world.

Chapter 1 What is 'health policy' and why do we need it?

In central and local government, policy is essentially a political process of decision-making. In certain public organisations – for example, those run as voluntary, charitable, not-for-profit bodies – policy may not be overtly political in the sense of following a particular ideological line. Nevertheless, underlying all policy are dominant *values*, that is the moral beliefs of those who have the authority to influence decisions in a political context. These value perspectives are said to range along a continuum from state non-intervention (*laissez-faire*) to substantial state intervention (socialism). In practice, the value system operating within the public sector generally, or within particular sections or institutions, will largely determine the manner in which policy comes to be changed.

In trying to understand how and why policy is formed for the provision of health services, it is often necessary to go to original sources of information such as transcripts of parliamentary speeches and debates, minutes of official meetings, official reports and government papers. However, it is also necessary on many occasions to consider other possible motives for generating policies in order to comprehend why a certain policy has been formulated and for what purpose. Some of the possible reasons for formulating a particular health or health care policy are given below. You may wish to add others:

- A desire to improve people's quality of life
- An attempt to improve a nation's competitiveness
- A perceived need to reduce costs or save money
- A perceived need to stabilise expenditure but improve the standard of services
- A pragmatic concern to retain power and authority.

What is 'policy'?

We shall not attempt to provide a definition of 'policy' because it may mean different things according to the context in which the word is used. However, there are certain attributes or characteristics of 'policy' that can be specified:

- 'Policy' denotes belongingness: a policy belongs to someone or some body. It is the government's policy – departmental policy or party policy, for example.
- 'Policy' denotes commitment. A stated intention, for example, is not merely a statement. Commitment implies a desire to 'see it through', to make sure that something happens.
- 'Policy' also has status; that is to say, it has the backing of a group of influential people such as a government or board of directors in a company.

Hogwood and Gunn (1984) in their book *Policy Analysis for the Real World*, have listed a number of ways in which the word 'policy' is used. We shall select what we think are the most significant and relevant for our purposes:

1. *Policy as aspiration or general purpose.* So-called mission statements come under this heading. These often state a position or value. 'We believe that the health of the nation is the first priority in terms of public spending' is one example of this use of the term 'policy'.
2. *Policy as one proposal or a set of proposals.* This is a more specific statement; for example, a government could declare its intention 'by the year 2010 to reduce the death rate from cancer amongst people aged under 65 years at least a further fifth'. (Consultation Paper 1998)
3. *Policy as a particular programme.* This will involve a 'package' or a statement of intended action focusing on a clearly identified group of people or on a type of health care intervention. For example, a government might set out proposals for a systematic health screening programme to detect breast cancer.
4. *Policy as formally authorised action.* This happens when a government, for example, states its intentions in a piece of legislation, a White Paper or a Charter, or when a health care organisation, such as a hospital, publishes its prospectus.

5. *Policy as a process.* We shall deal with this matter more fully in Chapter 3. For Hogwood and Gunn, 'process' refers to the progress of any policy from its original appearance on the 'agenda' to its eventual implementation, review and evaluation.

Health and health care policy

In this book, we shall be dealing almost exclusively with health care policy, which is policy relating to the professional intervention in people's lives at the prevention, promotion, maintenance, cure and rehabilitation stages. Health policy has a much broader remit and at a state or city or national level may involve several different departments, for example, environmental health, water and sewerage, housing and transport. This wider application is often referred to as 'public health policy' as opposed to 'health care policy'.

Two interpretations of health policy in the widest sense – that is, as including both 'public health' and 'health care' policy – can be considered:

1. An authoritative statement of intent adopted by governments on behalf of the public with the aim of improving the health and welfare of the population, that is, a centrally determined basis for action.
2. What health agencies actually do rather than what governments would like them to do. Health policy can only be determined by the observation of the outcomes of decision-making.

We shall note in Chapter 4 that the process of implementing policy is not always straightforward. People whose task it is to meet the public face to face might not want or be able to put into effect those policies which have been determined 'from above'. Lack of time, expertise or resources, for example, could militate against the full implementation of policies intended to reduce hospital waiting lists or create more opportunities for care in the community.

Policy as the 'rationalisation of values'

This acknowledgement of possible tensions between policy as stated and policy as enacted suggests that at the heart of all political decisions is the allocation of values. Easton, in 1965, developed a systems model in order to explain his interpretation of the policy-making process. In his model, inputs (demands, resources or support) were fed into the 'black box' of government institutions and then emerged as outputs (goods and services). For Easton, the allocation of values is the process by which governments choose which values to grant and which to deny – the process of making or altering policies. Governments, because of competing demands on finite resources, have to make choices.

- Demands are made by individuals or groups seeking particular policies, for example better care in the community, shorter waiting times for hospital admission or more money to be spent on research.
- Resources help the government to respond to the demands being made. Resources may include money, buildings, staff and time.
- Support relates to the extent to which any government is authorised to pass legislation. Support may be shown through the ballot box at times of elections, or a one-party system of government may, in effect, authorise its own policies.

Demands, resources and support are fed into Easton's 'black box' of policy-making and, as a result, policies are formulated, implemented and, if necessary, revised.

Can there be 'negative' policies?

We have so far mainly been talking about 'policy' as being positive, as both a statement involving values and, in its more specific form, as an intention to *do* something. However, it will be remembered that the idea of *laissez-faire* may also be applicable to a government's policy on health or any other social issue. In fact, the direct or indirect involvement of governments in providing health care is relatively recent compared with, for example, many countries' raising of revenue through taxes in order to fight against other countries. Foreign policy has been and still is a major concern for most developed and developing countries, and in the past, the need for a government to take action to improve people's health was prompted – as it is now – by a mixture of economic and political motives rather than by an exclusively humanitarian urge to help citizens to enjoy a healthier lifestyle.

In Britain, for example, the recruitment of potential soldiers to serve in the Boer War at the end of the nineteenth century revealed a poor state of health among a significant proportion of young men. Industrialists, too, were concerned about the poor health of employees and the consequent detrimental effect upon production. As Saville (1983) has remarked:

A labour force that suffers from a high incidence of disease – the result of dirt, poor housing, inadequate diet – is an inefficient labour force and therefore the improvement of the physical environment in which working people live, the means for purchasing an adequate food supply, the availability of medical services in sufficient quantity and at a satisfactory level of competence, are all necessary if the industrial machine is to work at full stretch. (p. 13)

The economic motive for improving public health status has been reaffirmed in the UK government's consultation paper *Our Healthier Nation* (DoH 1998):

There are sound economic reasons for improving our health. 187 million working days are estimated by industry to be lost every year because of sickness – a £12 billion tax on business. (p. 4)

Even though many people and pressure groups might firmly believe that action needs to be taken in order to make some improvement in health, a government might choose to do nothing. It might, in a way, formulate a policy of inaction. Controversial issues such as abortion and euthanasia are so fraught with ethical concerns that many governments might choose not to have any policies designed to lay down clear courses of action. This is because, in the field of health and health care, decisions often have to be made within a framework of competing values.

Potential roles for government in health care

One potential role, then, for a government in relation to health care provision is to adopt a stance of *laissez-faire*, that is, to avoid any direct intervention in policy and to let market forces determine who gets what and at what price. In this case, the government will, in one sense, be seen as advocating a positive policy approach in that it is openly stating its support for a market-driven economy in health care provision in which health is regarded as a commodity. In reality, it would be highly unlikely for any country to adopt a completely 'hands-off' approach to health care provision, not least because of the adverse political repercussions that such a policy would probably create. Many governments have become involved in at least one or two of the potential roles mapped out by Lee and Mills (1985), as:

- A regulator of health care agencies
- A stimulator of research
- A protector of deprived and disadvantaged groups
- A financier of health and health care programmes
- A purchaser of health care services
- A direct provider of services.

Even in those countries such as the USA and Singapore, which rely heavily on private and employer-financed insurance schemes to resource the health care system, subsidised provision is made for people on low incomes who cannot afford to pay the full cost of treatment. Even though, as in the USA, this public policy still leaves a large number of citizens without basic health care coverage, a considerable proportion of the total public expenditure is earmarked for the health care services. As can be noted in the typologies of health care systems developed by Field (1989), an 'emergent' health care system in which the state plays only a minimal role is not a model that can be readily ascribed to any particular country since nearly all governments take on some responsibility for enabling poorer citizens to have access to health care services.

- Type 1 – Emergent: health care viewed as an item of personal consumption; private ownership of facilities; physicians operate as solo entrepreneurs.

- Type 2 – Pluralistic: health care viewed mainly as a consumer good; private and public ownership of facilities; state's role in health care is minimal and indirect. (Example: USA.)
- Type 3 – Insurance/social security: health care seen as an insured/guaranteed consumer good or service; private and public ownership of facilities; payments for services are mostly indirect; state's role in health care is central but indirect. (Example: France.)
- Type 4 – National health service: health care viewed as a state-supported service; facilities mainly publicly owned; payments for services are indirect; state's role is central and direct. (Example: UK.)
- Type 5 – Socialised: health care seen as a state-provided service; physicians are state employees; facilities are wholly publicly owned; payments for services are entirely indirect; state's role in health care is total. (Example: former Soviet Union.)

The five types of health care system reproduced above depict *models* of systems that might not exist in their 'pure' form. In real life, a health care system might include certain attributes of more than one type, as in Belgium and Spain, where public expenditure on health care has increased considerably over the past three decades.

Dimensions of policy-making

In essence, a social problem is not a social problem unless those in power decide that the issue is worthy of attention. This preliminary process of 'deciding to decide' has been described as the 'issue filtration stage' in the policy-making process (Hogwood and Gunn, 1984). As we shall see in Chapter 2, the capacity to decide which items reach the political agenda is a key attribute of power. By no means all the decisions that are generated by governments and large organisations are made in the public arena. The screening of issues – usually made in these contexts by a relatively small inner circle of senior persons – is referred to by Lukes (1974) as 'hidden politics'.

Lee and Mills (1985), in their book *Policy Making and Planning in the Health Sector*, have stated that:

policy making is concerned with what is politically feasible and what is technically desirable. (p. 29)

That is, governments have to strike a balance between what ought ideally to be done and what it is possible to do. There are restrictions – sometimes political, sometimes financial, sometimes both – but policy-making is more complex than Lee and Mills suggest.

For example, policy-makers have to take account of at least four key considerations:

1. *Political pragmatism.* 'If we choose this option, is it likely to be popular or unpopular?' This concern will be particularly important in systems in which there is a diversity of political parties competing for votes.
2. *Ideological.* The policy will conform to the core commitments of the most powerful group, for example the belief in the virtues of capitalism, socialism, professionalism and managerialism as the basis for policy-making.
3. *Financial.* What are the economic considerations that need to be identified before policy is made?
4. *Moral.* What are the key values that underlie policy-making? Does the government value the principles of equality of access to health care; of social equity, that is equal treatment for people with similar needs; of viewing good health care as a commodity rather than a public responsibility?

Individual and state responsibility

Health can also be seen as a means towards some further objective such as economic competitiveness or decreased public expenditure, or as an end in itself. Commitment by governments to the notion of health as an end in itself are likely to refer to human rights, of which good health and access to the health care services is one example. This is the stance adopted by the World Health Organisation (WHO, 1978). However, although good health might be championed by governments and citizens as a basic human right, and therefore as an apparent end in itself, there is no doubt that a healthy person would also regard this desirable state as a means towards achieving a good quality of life because poor health is likely to inhibit the capacity to engage fully in <u>occupational, recreational and social activities</u>. In other words, *physical impairment* can result in *personal disability* and *social handicap,* as we shall note more fully in Chapter 8.

The moral issue may also be expressed in terms of *obligation* or *responsibility.* That is to say, governments may argue that it is the individual's responsibility to maintain a state of good health and that it is therefore morally irresponsible to adopt a lifestyle that is likely to incur unnecessary expense for a public health service. People, therefore, who smoke, drink to excess, take drugs or rarely take exercise may be seen as acting antisocially. The mandatory wearing of seat belts in cars and crash helmets for motor cyclists is accepted in many countries as a necessary intrusion on an individual's personal freedom because these restrictions help to reduce the number of deaths and serious injuries suffered in road accidents. A government imposing such mandatory measures will undoubtedly have regard to the consequent reduction in expenditure on medical treatment.

The focus of the chapters

Easton's model is useful as a conceptual tool but – as we shall see in Chapter 2 – we need to think more about issues of power and policy-making. How do various theories of power illuminate the actual process of decision-making in the real world? We also need to look, in Chapter 3, at criticisms of rational models of decision-making. For example, whether demands are listened to carefully by a government may depend on the political 'colour' of the pressure group, on whether the government considers the issue to be one that – for one reason or another – requires a positive response or one that can be ignored without any political repercussions.

Chapters 4 and 5 deal with policy implementation and policy evaluation as key components in the whole policy-making process. These stages – which are not to be construed as the final stages of decision-making but part of a cyclical process – are critical in order to assess the compatibility between policy objectives and policy outcomes. In order to provide a schema for analysing the extent to which policy is successful in its aims, a systems model is presented in Chapter 5. This model highlights the main features of health care systems in terms of inputs, process, outputs and outcomes.

The various purposes of health care planning are dealt with in Chapter 6. In particular, the problem of reconciling demand with resources features as a key issue, and reference to an early attempt in the USA to engage members of the public in planning introduces the question of whether or not lay persons ought to be more involved with health care planning at various levels of decision-making.

The debate widens in Chapter 7 to a discussion about the value of health care planning in terms of rationing and prioritising resources and resource allocation, and a number of critical perspectives are offered concerning the ways in which certain approaches to planning might disadvantage different groups of actual and potential service users.

The importance of applying reliable, accurate and comprehensive data, and of interpreting the data so that they yield useful information to assist the planning process, is the subject matter of Chapters 8 and 9. The contemporary debate about health care outcomes and evidence-based medical practice is presented as a central issue in developing more 'rational' bases for resource allocation decisions at central and devolved levels.

The final chapter draws attention to the probable areas of research and 'scenario-building' for health care policy and planning that are likely to occupy the minds of politicians, health care professionals and the public over the next few decades.

Summary

In this chapter, we have sketched out the various interpretations of the term 'policy' and looked at a number of reasons why a government or an organisation should feel a need to devise policies in respect of health care. We have highlighted the complex balancing act that the policy-makers will have to perform, and have also noted that policy-makers have the option of doing nothing if they consider that action in relation to any particular health issue is not justified. Policy-making is essentially a political enterprise that is founded on the dominant values of policy-makers within a particular social context. Although the emphasis has, in this chapter, been on policy-making at central government level, the main concerns to be raised in subsequent chapters are equally relevant to health care organisations such as primary care agencies, hospitals and community care services in the statutory, private and not-for-profit sectors.

Items for discussion

1. You might wish to consider which of the four 'dimensions' of policy-making – political pragmatism and ideological, moral and political concerns – are likely to be uppermost in the minds of politicians in developed countries when they decide to offer material help to less wealthy countries.
2. Consider the question of which rights and responsibilities might be influential in determining a government's commitment to providing public funds for various health care services.

Chapter 2 Power and policy-making

In Chapter 1 we referred to 'values' as being a key consideration in the process of policy-making. To reinforce this point, we can talk about a 'value system' as:

the moral principles in which policy is embedded, a prevailing ideology based on beliefs about what is worthy – a vision of the most desirable society.

These principles may not always be made explicit in policy state- ments. When reading about health and health care policy, it may be necessary to adopt a critical approach and ask ourselves, On what value system is this particular policy based?

Easton's (1965) model of the political system identified values as a key input and the allocation of values as a function of govern- ment. Allocating values may seem a strange idea, but it essentially means that governments are granted power or assume power in order to run a country according to certain ideological beliefs about what is right and wrong for a particular society. Where the value systems of a government and its citizens are at one – where there is little discord or disagreement about what ought to happen – creating and implementing social policy, health policy and any other kind of policy will present few problems other than the perennial one of finite resources: choices will always have to be made between competing claims for expenditure.

Different models of power

Much of the literature that deals with issues of power and policy- making derives from a particular cultural setting. Texts written by academics in the USA and the UK are almost unavoidably ethnocentric, that is to say, they do not look beyond their own country in arriving at decisions about how power issues affect policy-making. It is important to remember this and, if necessary, to challenge such models as being perhaps of limited applicability to other countries. Certainly, the word 'model' is not being used here in the sense of some ideal type of system that everyone ought to try to follow. The word 'theory' is sometimes used in academic and other texts when 'model' would be a more accurate representation of an attempt to explain phenomena by using distinct conceptual frameworks.

Various models are presented in the literature, offering a framework within which to analyse the process of policy-making. The fact is that, in the field of social policy, no single model or theory is able to explain how every policy decision comes to be shaped and formulated. Each model or theory has something to offer in the way of interpretation. We must remember, however, that there will be exceptions depending on the particular circumstances of time and location in which the policy is being drawn up.

Hypotheses, concepts, models and theories

Hypotheses

Hypotheses are tentative statements asserting a relationship between certain facts, to be tested empirically and either verified or rejected. Hypotheses are derived from a theoretical system and the results of past research. There are different kinds of hypotheses. Perhaps the most familiar is the causal hypothesis – the 'if... then' statement. To be acceptable as an hypothesis a statement must be

- Derived from a firmer base than merely one's own experience
- Capable of being tested empirically.

Example

> Research evidence might indicate that the great majority of elderly people prefer to remain living in their own homes for as long as possible. If this finding is based on a limited range of survey-type data, the assertion could be used as an hypothesis to be tested further.

Concepts

A concept is not 'discoverable'; it is a mental construct that is a means of classifying empirical phenomena. The use of concepts is selective and may, therefore, reflect a certain point of view or interpretation of data.

Example

> The concept of the mortification of self, derived from Goffman's (1968) observation of asylum inmates in the USA, has been influential in the move away from institutional care settings towards a greater emphasis on community services for people with mental health problems. Other concepts currently informing the debate about the provision of community care services include 'empowerment', 'citizenship' and 'welfare pluralism'.

Concepts are not strictly definable. They reflect the values of those who attempt to order a diversity of phenomena, and derive from and influence an individual's perception of 'reality'.

Models

A model is an attempt to systematise patterns observed in the world of social behaviour. Models, although partial and tentative, are the building blocks of theory.

Example

> Drawing upon the concept of consumerism, models may be devised of
>
> 1. Token consumerism
> 2. Participative consumerism
> 3. Controlling consumerism.
>
> These and other models help to assign order to an interpretation of social behaviour by ascribing particular aspects of that observed behaviour to a distinct classifiable group.

Theory

Theories attempt to explain a wide variety of phenomena. A theory consist of a set of logically interrelated, empirically verifiable propositions. These propositions may be regarded as *laws* if they have been sufficiently verified to be widely accepted or as *hypotheses* if they have not been that well verified.

In either case, the propositions that constitute a theory are constantly subjected to further empirical testing and revision. Sociological theory, for example, attempts to provide systematic explanations and predictions relating to human social interaction. Early originators of theory in this field were Weber (1948), Mead (1934) and Durkheim (1938).

Examples

> The Marxist theory concerning the principles of social interaction posits a world in which materialist interests are pursued in a capitalist world of contradiction, for example between private appropriation and socialised production (Marx, 1867). Another sociological theory is functionalism, which perceives an analogy between biology and social structure and process. The perception of the world as being analogous to a system akin to a controllable engineered mechanism is another example of a theoretical framework designed to organise selected aspects of the observable social world.
>
> Like models, theories are partial explanations of phenomena that need to be compared with broadly conflicting or compatible theories in order to test their adequacy.

Summary

Thus, *concepts* help build *models*, which help to construct *theories*, which help to state *laws*.

Models of power

The consensus model

Power is granted to governments by the people through periodic elections. The government then pursues policies in the common interest of everyone in society. The view of power in this model is that power is positive or at least neutral. This model assumes that nearly everyone agrees on the key goals to be achieved for society at large, that there is a harmony of interests. It is a very clear and uncomplicated view of how society works and how political decisions are made, and it has been criticised for presenting too 'rationalist' an interpretation of power. Talcott Parsons (1967), in *Sociological Theory and Modern Society*, was the most influential writer who put forward this consensus model of power.

The pluralist model

The text by Walt (1994) discusses other models of power in some detail. Here, we shall summarise the main points. The pluralist view is that no one group holds total power. Citizens have rights to elect who will be the government, pressure groups act on behalf of ordinary people, and opposition political parties are able to express their contesting ideas about what ought to be done. The state neither defends the interests of any one particular class or group, nor shows bias towards particular interests. This view is, however, really a modified version of the consensus model, and although it recognises that there are powerful groups pressing their claims for policies to be enacted that will favour their positions, the pluralist perception of power distribution is that harmony is maintained by the government as a kind of neutral negotiator.

Critics of this model argue that most governments listen more attentively to those pressure groups whose interests coincide with the ideological standpoint of the party in power. Trades unions, for example, are likely to be influential in policy-making when a left-wing government is in control; conversely, groups representing the interests of business and commerce put their weight behind more right-wing administrations and may contribute to a political party's funds.

The élitist model

Karl Marx (1867) provided the core argument against the view that there is a general consensus in societies about value systems and that governments act as 'honest brokers', reconciling the competing interests of different groups towards agreed goals. He maintained that dominant social classes held the ultimate power to serve their own interests and suppress less powerful social classes. In many countries, there is evidence that a relatively small circle of businessmen, professionals, military leaders and politicians holds the real power. Later, Althusser (1971) and Gramsci (1971) stressed the influence of the media shaping the structures of power.

The élitist view holds that not all interest groups are equally powerful or influential. In the health field, for example, tobacco and pharmaceutical industries exert a powerful influence in many countries over health policy or, in effect, the absence of policy. In the interests of general health standards, governments have the power to place a complete ban on the sale and consumption of cigarettes. However, it is unlikely that policies will ever go this far, not because it would be seen as an infringement of personal liberties – after all, the wearing of car seat belts is compulsory in many countries – but because the huge revenue from the sale of cigarettes would be lost to the Treasury. Not all groups enjoy the same degree of power in the health care sector, where the doctors' influence usually dominates the interests of nurses, paramedics and patients. A further challenge to the pluralist and consensus models is that, in today's world, the influence of multinational corporations, and of political and trade alliances between countries, often guides domestic policy.

Perhaps some sort of compromise could be agreed: that on 'grand issues' such as defence and international trade and finance, powerful élite groups would exercise considerable power to influence strategic policy-making. In other, more domestic, areas of policy, such as transport, education and health, government might fulfil a role that comes close to that of a mediator, resolving or heading off potential or actual conflicts of interest through discussion and negotiation with a variety of interest groups.

Policy networks

In the field of health care, several organisations might have to collaborate in order to plan a co-ordinated assessment and provision of services. This would be particularly appropriate in deciding the most cost-effective method of delivering services in community settings. In such cases, the establishment of policy networks at 'subgovernment' level (Gray 1994) would operate at both a formal and an informal level across agencies. Flynn *et al.* (1996) concluded, from the results of several case studies focusing on purchasing and providing functions within the British NHS, that the whole enterprise depended on interagency and interprofessional collaboration founded on mutual trust. This conclusion supports the results of research by Granovetter (1985), who identified the importance of *social* networks between firms who were ostensibly in competition with each other.

In an ideal world, these policy networks would always work smoothly together and in line with central government policy. Gray (1994), however, points out that even when central government appears to have a clear picture of what a policy should be achieving, the role of the organisations who actually deliver the services gives them the opportunity to modify or otherwise adapt this picture to fit in more comfortably with their own preferences. An example of this proposition is the provision of community care, which relies upon a network of health, social services and housing agencies to implement the overall policy at ground level. Gray maintains that 'the more homogeneous or tightly-knit the organisational community that is involved in the policy area, the less likely it is that disagreement about policy will take place' (pp. 126–7).

Lukes and power

Steven Lukes (1974) regards many of the theories and models of power as being rather naïve and unrelated to the real world of politics. He offers what he calls the 'second and third dimensions of power'. In his interpretation of how decisions are made at government level, he makes the following assertions:

1. Policy is shaped by political leaders in conjunction with other 'élite' group representatives. Although nominally accountable to the public at large, such power-holders manipulate the policy-making process in order to legitimise their own position.
2. The executive, for example the civil servants, side with the élite power-holders. Far from being an impartial agency, the

executive/administration will either support vested interests or even play a proactive role in policy-making.

3. There is an imbalance of power, resources and skills in society, which means that industrial and corporate interests, or government interests, usually dominate weaker or less well-resourced groups. The more powerful groups control the policy agenda, suppressing information about contentious issues and deciding in various ways not to act on them.

4. Although there is in some countries public debate that is open to the media, the most important decisions are taken secretly. At both local and regional and central government levels, the main political party will usually meet as a group before key issues are to be discussed in order to 'orchestrate' the debate – rather like a dress rehearsal for a dramatic performance – and decide who will speak, who will ask which questions and what the eventual outcome of the vote will be. In his interpretation, Lukes is essentially writing about 'hidden politics' – what goes on behind the scenes and out of public view.

Lukes' 'third dimension of power' relates to the impact of ideological principles on policy. Ideology shapes the way in which social issues are seen by those in power, and their view, in turn, shapes the way these issues are seen by the general population. Navarro (1978) has argued along similar lines – that despite many health problems having their root cause in political and economic circumstances, the medical profession has successfully transmitted the prevailing view that ailments are best treated on an individual physician–patient basis.

Foucault (1973) also has asserted that powerful élites are able to shape public desires by imposing upon society their own particular perspectives and definitions. The dominance of the medical profession during the twentieth century has, it is argued, resulted in the medicalisation of health policy to an oppressive extent. According to this thesis, a wide variety of physical and mental disorders have become subject to clinical diagnosis and treatment despite the fact that medical knowledge is deficient in many areas of so-called expertise. Marinker (1994), a medical practitioner and academic, has referred to 'the profound uncertainties and ambiguities in medicine that masquerade as facts' (p. 3).

Illich (1975) also takes issue with what he considers to be the unjustified power of the medical profession and argues that, far from deserving this élite position in society, clinicians are at times a threat to the health and well-being of individuals and of societies. The administration of drugs that have had serious side-effects, the incidence of hospital-induced infections and examples of medical negligence all testify to the unfounded elevation of the medical profession to a status of social pre-eminence. Furthermore, in the view of Illich and of Zola (1975), the medical labels attached to a wide range of social and individual problems have given the medical profession an enormous power to judge others. Moves to increase consumer involvement in health care decisions and to impose a more rational organisation of health care services will, according to Illich, prove ineffective in reducing medical power. The only real solution will be to limit the scope of professional monopolies and to extend personal responsibility for health.

Various stake-holders in health care systems

Governments will, of course, try to base policies on their value systems; a commitment, for example, to the principles of capitalism, of socialism or of liberalism will steer policies in the direction of what those in power regard as the 'best society'. In many cases, however, policy-making demands negotiation and compromise. When the socialist government in Britain, after the Second World War ended in 1945, was attempting to establish a National Health Service for everyone free at the point of need, the government of the day met fierce opposition from the medial profession. Doctors did not want to become state employees; they wished to retain their autonomy as self-employed practitioners and also wanted to retain the right to treat patients privately at their surgeries or in hospitals. In order to make headway on their proposals, the government had to give in. Ironically, when the Conservative government, which held office in Britain from 1979 to 1997, wished to revamp the NHS in order to create a form of competition by making public hospitals compete for patients, the British Medical Association was its most stern opponent in its resolve to prevent the fragmentation of a health service still largely free at the point of service delivery. The NHS remained intact, but GPs were given the opportunity to become fund-holders in order to purchase health care on behalf of their patients. Certain commentators recognised, in health care policies at this time, a concern to replace some of the power and authority of the medical profession – a dominant group – with a new emphasis on the development of an emerging group: health care managers (Harrison and Pollitt 1994).

The advent of *managerialism* within various health care systems testifies to a move away from total professional hegemony towards an organisational system that recognises the desirability of appointing non-medical experts as the senior executives within health care organisations. In Britain, for example, the chief executive officer of multi-million pound health service Trusts is just as likely to be an accountant as a medically trained official. The business entrepreneur and the economist are also becoming important contributors to health care planning decisions. In an era of increasing demand on health care resources throughout the developed and developing countries of the world, the criterion of clinical efficacy in assessing the calibre of health care is now being supplemented by the criteria of efficiency, equity, accessibility, acceptability and appropriateness (Maxwell 1984). Value for money and public accountability, linked to a drive for total quality management (TQM), relate to criteria that recognise the need for effective resource management and public accountability, and also clearly acknowledge the variety of interest groups that health services in the public and private sectors have to serve.

Who does and who should influence health and health care policy?

Before discussing this question, it is important to distinguish between three levels of decision-making:

1. *Strategic*:   broad policy, long-term 'legislative'
2. *Operational*:   managing, administering, implementing, 'executive'
3. *Practitioner*: ground level, face to face, 'grass roots'.

Traditionally, politicians, through their role in government, make decisions and create policy at the strategic level, civil servants and perhaps other agencies such as voluntary bodies and local government act as the executive arm of government, while professionals make decisions that will directly affect the client/patient.

There are, however, movements in many countries to alter the balance of power within these three categories of policy. For example, 'consumer' is replacing the notion of 'patient', in line with the development of a more market-orientated model of health care systems. In the UK over the past 20 years, since a major reorganisation of the NHS, the government has placed emphasis on the need to appoint managers in key hospital or 'Trust' organisations. The former dominant position of doctors is under scrutiny since 'the new managerialism' and 'consumerism' have begun to have an effect upon the deployment of resources. The three Es – economy, efficiency and effectiveness – have become crucial concerns for the providers, whether public or private, of many health care systems.

One important issue is who should assess the 'success' of health care in terms of these three criteria. Should doctors and/or service users and/or the general public become involved in:

- Determining objectives, priorities and standards
- Allocating resources
- Reviewing performances against objectives
- Reviewing the objectives?

We shall deal more extensively with these questions in Chapter 6.

In terms of the capacity to influence decisions in the arena of health services, Alford (1975) described three types of what he termed 'structural interests'. These do not have to be organised into 'interest groups' in order to present demands or grievances to the appropriate authorities. The three types of structural interest are dominant, challenging and repressed.

Dominant structural interests

An example of a dominant structural interest is that found in a professional monopoly such as medical practitioners who, through their organised associations, exert control over who may or may not enter the profession according to prescribed qualifications. Alford (1975) contests the orthodox view that it is the high esteem in which physicians are held that enables them to influence the content of legislation and the actual implementation of policy:

Rather than a societal consensus giving the doctors power, it is the doctors' power which generates the societal consensus... the existence of a network of political, legal and economic institutions which guarantees that certain dominant interests will be served comes to be taken for granted as legitimate, as the only possible way in which these health services can be provided. People come to accept as inevitable that which exists and even believe that it is right. But this is quite a different argument from the one which says that because people believe in doctors, they give them power. (p. 17)

Challenging structural interests

Challenging structural interests include a range of health administrators, managers and researchers who are challenging the fundamental interests of professional monopolies and exerting increasing influence over the production and distribution of health care.

Repressed structural interests

Repressed structural interests are those of the 'community population', who are relatively poor and marginalised but who can organise into an interest group in order to strive for better health care facilities.

Until recently, patients have been suffering from a repressed structural interest. The very word 'patient' has as its root meaning 'to endure; to bear; to be long-suffering', and it has clear semantic associations with being 'passive'. Yet, in the 1980s and 90s, in line with an international orientation towards consumerism, patients – now redesignated 'service users' or even 'customers' – members of the public, have come to be regarded as potentially significant contributors to health care policy and planning, at least at certain levels of decision-making. Patients' charters, patient satisfaction surveys, opportunities for lodging complaints, representation on hospital and health authority boards – many of these developments in Britain have their counterparts in European, American and Asian health care systems outside the private sector. It remains to be seen whether erstwhile disempowered patients and the lay public generally will exert any significant influence on the direction and resourcing of health care systems.

Degrees of involvement in policy-making

If we take the analogy with the marketplace and apply it to the arena of health care, we may have a clearer picture of whether the increased involvement of ordinary people in strategic, operational and practitioner decisions is a wholly desirable objective. Basically, consumers who buy goods can enjoy various rights, which are set out in laws, charters and regulations. They have a right to redress, for example, if the merchandise is faulty: they can have goods replaced or get their money back, and/or receive monetary compensation.

They also have a right, within the limits of their financial circumstances, to shop elsewhere. In a mixed economy of care in which there is a degree of competition between the providers of health services, it is argued that people have the *choice* of where they wish to go for assistance. This right is often called the 'right of exit'.

Consumers are sometimes also invited to contribute towards decisions concerning the design, specifications and standards of goods and services. They have a *voice*, which can be expressed as part of a marketing research survey, as a company share-holder or as an individual complainant, for example. Yet, even in the marketplace, ordinary citizens do not often sit on boards of directors, and it is questionable whether people necessarily desire the level of influence that certain politicians, academics and other advocates of citizen power claim that they should have.

Consumerism and empowerment

Ransom and Stewart (1994) have argued that 'consumerism provides an incomplete and ultimately inadequate language for the public domain' (p. 19). They point out that public organisations have the task of exercising the powers of the state; sometimes they have to order, inspect and control, and public bodies often have to ration or prioritise services, determining who shall and shall not receive them. In the public domain, public purposes have to be realised that may not conform to the wishes of individual members of the public. For example, the allocation of housing to ex-mental health patients might be strenuously opposed by local residents. Furthermore, the 'consumer' or 'customer' might be the community at large. Action taken to improve the environment is intended positively to affect the health of whole neighbourhoods, often over a wide geographical area. Following on from this line of debate, it could be argued that the planned improvement of individual health status by governments is motivated by the need in the long term to reduce public expenditure on health care services. In this case, the consumer as key beneficiary is the government itself. In other words, policy statements linked to an ideological commitment to enhance choice for individuals appear to conflict with equally pressing commitments to plan for the health needs of local populations. This potential dilemma will come into clearer focus in Chapter 6, where we shall consider certain policy initiatives concerning the allocation of public resources in health care. Decisions about who shall and who shall not receive treatment at public expense raise serious ethical concerns in which the individual's interests and the collective interests of society at large have to be weighed in the balance.

Key words in the lexicon of consumerism are 'empowerment' and 'choice'. These can easily become rather empty slogans unless they embody an unambiguous resolve to adjust the balance of power between sections of society. In the health care field, as in any other area of individual and social welfare, ideological conviction is liable to submerge reality under a sea of untested assumptions. There is a rather piquant irony inherent in many political statements advocating citizen choice and empowerment in that little or no consultation may have taken place with the public, as the intended beneficiaries, over what form or extent of choice and empowerment they would regard as desirable.

The idea that a consensus can be reached about such matters is also debatable. Holland and Blackburn (1998) point out that empowerment often threatens vested interests and that such threats create conflict. Participatory approaches to decision-making also challenge 'the myth of the homogeneous "community"' (p. 193), an issue of concern to Braye and Preston-Shoot (1995), who refer to the need to acknowledge cultural pluralism. People from different ethnic groups and religious backgrounds, for example, might express quite different expectations of empowerment and choice.

In an extensive analysis of the different concepts and interpretations of 'empowerment', Servian (1996, p. 8) draws attention to the definitive statement by the Audit Commission in relation to the principles informing the NHS and Community Care Act 1990 in Britain:

The first aim (of the community care legislation) is to empower the service users and their carers.

Servian's findings from research carried out in one region of England showed that service users' interpretation of 'empowerment' related to getting support when they needed it (*responsiveness* and *accessibility*), to their wishes being taken seriously (*empathy* and *sincerity*), and to access to information and facilities kept from them by petty rules made by managers and administrators (*real communication* and *access*). Certainly, it is difficult to make general statements about the preferred choices and examples of empowerment that would appeal to all service users. Decisions of this kind are likely to depend on individuals within a particular context.

For example, soon after the implementation of the NHS and Community Care Act, the author was invited to act as external evaluator of a quality action group set up by a social services department in a purpose-built residential and day centre for disabled people. The fact that the centre had been designed without consulting any disabled persons is, in itself, an example of disempowerment. However, in the spirit of the new national policy of 'consumerism', representatives of middle management explained to a hand-picked group of service users, their staff and volunteer helpers that they were to be offered more choices about their use of the centres.

To summarise the findings, disabled people started to push the boundaries of management expectations concerning legitimate areas of choice – which day(s) to attend the day centre, greater choice of food at meal-times – towards more meaningful choices such as contributing to decisions about staff appointments and choosing which member of staff should be their key worker. During the early part of this innovative policy initiative, agenda-setting, in its literal and metaphorical senses, was performed 'from above'. For the remainder of the evaluation period, professionals and disabled people manoeuvred to negotiate adjustments to what might be termed, in the analysis by Lukes (1974), the 'structured imbalance of power'.

Empowerment and choice in action can be analysed along a number of dimensions:

- The levels of decision-making in which users are involved
- The nature of that involvement
- The identifiable contribution of service users in terms of the decisions made
- The range of decision-making made accessible to service users.

The most crucial of the four is perhaps 'the nature of involvement' for, as Arnstein (1969) demonstrated in the context of community development projects in the USA, expressions of apparently people-centred policies, for example 'participation' and 'consultation', can often be deceptive.

Arnstein's 'ladder'

Arnstein (1969) presents in diagrammatic form various degrees of citizen participation in decision-making. The eight levels can be used as a useful analytical tool in order to evaluate the nature of citizen involvement in health care policy-making and planning. The two elements that comprise the lowest level, that of *non-participation*, attract the pejorative labels of 'manipulation' and 'therapy', the latter indicating a concept akin to 'brainwashing'. At this level, lay people might be said to be 'involved' with decision-making only in the sense that they are being used in order to approve of decisions already made by powerful interest groups and/or individuals. The term 'tokenism' epitomises a number of activities that give the appearance of genuine citizen participation in a democratic decision-making process, but which offer no guarantee that the views of patients or their families, or of the public at large, will influence the final decisions. 'Consultation', for example, could feature in the next level, *participation*, if it meant that the process actually did contribute to decisions.

One of the most deceptive strategies for managing the illusion of citizen participation is *placation*. This occurs, for example, when an ex-mental health patient is co-opted onto a relatively high-level committee in order to represent the viewpoint of all such former patients in a particular locality. Without the power of veto, one individual is clearly unlikely to exert much influence on the outcome of committee meetings where he or she can be out-voted by a considerable margin.

At the highest level in Arnstein's model of citizen participation – partnership – ordinary citizens have an increasingly influential role to play. It could be argued that partnership might not entail a very evenly balanced allocation of power since, in reality, partners in various enterprises might play more dominant or relatively submissive roles. This could well occur in the context of community mental health teams and other collaborative bodies set up to co-ordinate health care services. There is evidence to suggest that such bodies are often 'partnerships' only in the most limited sense. Ovretveit *et al.* (1997), drawing upon the findings of many years of research in the field of inter-agency collaboration, distinguish between equal and unequal 'partnerships':

When a number of people from different disciplines come together, each used to working in different structures and having different expectations, it is not surprising if members in various ways come to feel that their contribution is not given the status they think it deserves. Interprofessional practice is not, however, to do with hierarchy of role or hierarchy of importance; it is a partnership in which everyone's contribution is of equal importance and each person has a distinctive role to play. (pp. 123–4)

Arnstein's model was used initially to illustrate the democratic deficit operating at federal and state level in the arena of community development in parts of the USA. It carries with it an ideological commitment to greater control by ordinary citizens over their environment and their standard of living. The potential hazard in applying this model to the analysis of public involvement in decision-making is that it might be prone to adopting a paternalistic approach by imposing on others its own ideological assumptions. As we have noted earlier, one important element in attempting to extend a wider range of choices for the consumers of health services is to give people the opportunity to decide what kind of choice they wish to make and in which circumstances they would wish to exercise that choice.

A simpler version of Arnstein's 'ladder' (Ham 1981), which ignores the significant elements of real power such as control over decisions, lists four types of citizen participation:

1. *Negotiation:* decisions depend largely on the group's approval
2. *Consultation:* the views of citizen groups may or may not be taken into account

3. *Public relations:* views are sought but will have no influence on decision-making
4. *Articulation:* the group presents its views without being asked.

Opportunities for ordinary people to play a substantial role in particular aspects of health care systems will be discussed in Chapters 5–9.

Summary

The need to analyse theories of power in order to understand the policy-making process has been highlighted in this chapter. We have noted that policy is fundamentally a political concern and that policy may be expressed as either a positive course of action or a decision to take no action. Power is also exercised in the setting of agendas, both literally and metaphorically, as élite groups and inner cabals determine what should occupy their minds as policy-makers. Although elected or self-appointed national leaders and their political in-groups exert primary control over policy-making, it must not be forgotten that their advisers – often senior civil servants – may also have a strong influence over what issues require a decision because they have access to information and can communicate or withhold such information in their own or in the national interest. The role of policy advisers or policy analysts is a feature of the next chapter. They have an increasingly important part to play in the health care policy process.

Finally, the potential contribution by the public to decision-making has been discussed with reference to the key concepts of *consumerism, empowerment* and *choice*. While there are compelling reasons for enabling potential and actual patients and the general public to become more directly engaged in decision-making at various levels, the point has been made that the imposition of ideologically motivated arguments needs to be avoided if people are going to assume powers and responsibilities that *they* would choose to enjoy.

Key Concepts in Health Care Policy and Planning

Items for discussion

1. To what extent does Alford's depiction of different structural interests influencing decisions apply to the health care systems with which you are familiar?
2. What would you consider to be the potential advantages and disadvantages of the public's involvement in decisions about where health care resources should go?

Chapter 3 Models of the policy process

In the previous two chapters, we attempted to deal with the following questions:

1. What is 'policy', and why are health care policies necessary?
2. Who makes policy and who *should* make policy?

In this chapter we need to describe *how* policy is made. To do this, we need to consider a number of models of the policy-making process and to clarify the distinction between analysis *of* policy and analysis *for* policy.

The role of the policy analyst is central to the process of policy-making. Governments and large organisations in both the public and private sectors rely on expert advice in order to help the policy-makers – that is those who have the power and authority to generate policies – to make key decisions. These advisers may be employed on a permanent basis or brought into the decision-making process at particular times, usually when particularly important decisions need to be made.

Clearly, at central and local government levels, civil servants and local government officers are continuously producing reports that are designed to assist politicians in their role as representative of the people. In profit-making companies, a core of senior employees will play a central part in feeding information to management so that decisions are based on information rather than hunches or mere past experience. These employees and special advisers hired using a contractual, fee-paid arrangement are often referred to as policy analysts. Their role is analysis *for* policy-making, analysis of present and future scenarios, analysis of trends and current information in a particular field of activity, analysis of various options and, perhaps, recommendations on the most favourable option to choose.

At what one might call the other end of the policy-making process, a great deal of time may be spent by a variety of interested people – such as academics, journalists, civil servants and politicians – in analysing policies that have already been created. We can call this activity the analysis *of* policy. These two activities must not, however, be regarded as quite distinct fields of enquiry because we can anticipate that government advisers will bring to their analysis for policy lessons learned from the past. In this way, the analysis *of* policy will contribute to the analysis *for* policy.

Since, however, policy-making, particularly at central government level, has to take account of not only what is feasible, but also what is politically and morally sound and what can be accomplished within a certain budget, the process of policy-making is likely to be complex and often time-consuming. Because decisions are frequently made 'behind closed doors', as Lukes (1974) suggests, this does not necessarily mean that there will be no disputes, disagreements and dissension even within the same political group. At local government level, especially where the elected members of an authority represent different political parties, the controlling faction will meet before key meetings in order to decide on the agenda, which items will be supported and which opposed, often by which speakers, so that the eventual meeting will have been 'orchestrated' well in advance and the public performance played out as a symbolic ritual of democratic debate.

In order to understand this process, a number of writers have set out models that are intended to identify what actually happens and/or what ought to happen when issues requiring policy decisions are considered. We shall now deal with these models of the policy-making process.

Comprehensive and bounded rationality

Several decades ago, Simon (1957) wrote about a model of the policy-making process that set out a highly rational, step-by-step analysis of how policy is made:

- First decide on the values that will guide the policy.
- Decide on the goals to be achieved by the policy.
- Search for possible means to achieve the goals.
- Evaluate each set of means or options.
- Select the 'best' option and implement it.

The test of a 'good' policy is that it can be shown to be the most appropriate means to the desired ends.

This clear distinction between the two processes of clarifying the desired ends and selecting the most suitable means for achieving them has been vividly presented in the structured approach to policy-making described by Patton and Sawicki (1986):

- *Step 1 – Identify and define the issue or problem.*
- *Step 2 – Establish evaluation criteria*, for example effectiveness, political acceptability, social equity or cost–benefit.
- *Step 3 – Identify alternative policies.* By whatever means are considered appropriate, suggest different ways of reaching the agreed goals/objectives. This might involve 'brainstorming', drawing on research findings. This prediction stage is technically quite difficult, and it is here that the policy analyst has to take into account possible political, economic and social scenarios.
- *Step 4 – Evaluate each alternative policy.* This step is vital. It involves a listing of the points in favour and against each of the proposals. This may demand different quantitative and qualitative techniques.
- *Step 5 – Display and select between alternative policies.* The results of Step 4 are presented for policy-makers to weigh up the preferred options. None of the alternatives will be perfect, but some may have potentially more politically/economically/socially better or worse outcomes than others.
- *Step 6 – Monitor policy outcomes.* There may be unintended consequences, poor implementation or changes in circumstances. This step will measure the impact that the policy is intended to have and whether the policy should be continued, modified or terminated.

Atkinson and Moon (1994) have produced a similar framework for policy analysis including nine components of the policy-making process.

Presented in this highly logical, carefully sequenced way, Simon's model of the policy process would seem to rely on a political consensus and little or no ideological conflict. Although highly rational, it does not allow for what might be called competing rationalities, that is, alternative and quite legitimate views about what the 'best' options are and, indeed, whether the desired ends are, in fact, justified. The issue arises, therefore, of the possible variance in different stake-holders' opinions of what is the most desirable and feasible course of action. Even a strictly top-down approach to policy-making, in which only the most powerful élite groups control the process of decision-making, may involve bargaining, negotiation and eventual compromise between the members of those groups. We have already noted two instances of these dynamics in Chapter 2 with regard to the formation and reformation of the NHS in Britain.

In the light of criticisms of this model, Simon acknowledged that a comprehensive, rational model might not reflect the real world and that policy-makers often have to make compromises between what they would consider to be the 'best' option and what is, in fact, possible to achieve. This anticipates the comment from Lee and Mills (1985) that 'policy-making is concerned both with what is politically feasible and what is technically desirable' (p. 29). In other words, policy-makers have to try to balance a keen ideological commitment with other pressing concerns such as the financial implications of policy and of potential political repercussions.

Simon, therefore, modified his *prescriptive* model – a model that depicted what ought to happen – with a more *descriptive* or real-life version. He named his revised model one of 'bounded rationality', the term 'bounded' meaning 'restrained' or 'limited'. According to this model, policy-makers often have to make do with a next best option, an option that will be good enough. Compressing the two words 'satisfy' and 'suffice', Simon coined a new term – 'satisfice' – to describe more accurately the policy-making process. He still maintained that rationality is essentially procedural, that is to say, that it may be viewed as selecting goals and courses of action that will best achieve the chosen values or purposes, and he distinguished between 'economic man' and 'administrative man':

While economic man maximises – selects the best alternative among all those available to him, his cousin, whom we shall call administrative man, satisfices – looks for a course of action that is satisfactory or 'good enough'. (Simon, 1957, p. 198)

Incrementalism

Writing in 1959, Lindblom presented a model that departs radically from that of Simon. According to Lindblom's analysis, policy at various levels is not made in some quasi-linear progression from issue identification through to policy implementation and review. He saw the process as being far more gradual and as arising out of previous policies limiting the amount of change that could be made.

Political, organisational, economic and situational (that is, the past, vested interests) constraints limit a purely 'rational' approach. Different power groups have an input into the policy process, and ultimately a system of partisan mutual adjustment has to be formed when those interested parties – perhaps the government, pressure groups, trade unions or political opposition parties – give ground in order to reach a mutually acceptable decision. In this way, policy is made by a process of muddling through; decisions are provisional, reviews continuous and errors eradicated 'en route'. Instead of some linear progression, as set out in Simon's models, the policy-makers are – according to Lindblom – likely to take two steps forwards and one step back on their way towards policy implementation.

Decision-making, in terms of 'muddling through', exhibits the following characteristics:

- It proceeds through incremental change.
- It involves mutual adjustment and negotiation.
- It excludes options by accident rather than by systematic or deliberate exclusion.
- Policy is not made once and for all.
- It proceeds through a series of incremental changes.
- The test of a good decision is agreement rather than meeting objectives.
- It involves trial and error.

In respect of the trial-and-error characteristic, Lindblom further depicted his model as a form of *disjointed incrementalism*, decisions not being subject to some overall plan or co-ordination.

This approach to policy-making was, in fact, advocated by a key adviser to Margaret Thatcher when, in the early 1980s, she announced a radical review of the NHS. She was advised by the American economist Alain Enthoven to test out the proposal for a purchaser–provider split among the health authorities and hospitals in a particular region in the UK and, in the light of that pilot project, to review the policy and take the appropriate action to implement, revise or shelve it. Enthoven returned from the USA to discover that his advice had not been heeded and that the government was going ahead and introducing major changes in the way in which the NHS was organised, notably by the creation of an internal market in which health authorities and GPs were empowered to purchase health care services from newly designated NHS Trusts. His remark made in a television account of this particular policy was that 'back home we don't go for the Big Bang policy-making'.

Critiques of both models

We must remember, when reading any literature relating to the policy-making process, that the ideas are rooted in a particular socio-cultural context and that while, for example Lindblom's model might seem relevant to the USA in the late 1950s and even today, it is not necessary applicable to all countries at all times.

Both Simon's and Lindblom's models may appear – in some other contexts – to be too 'cosy'. The representation of different interest groups reaching mutual agreement through a process of negotiation and bargaining is certainly not a worldwide descriptive model. In some situations, at certain times and in other countries, policy may be the result of a major 'climb-down' by the most powerful group in the face of serious and potentially disruptive confrontation.

In other countries where there is virtually one-party rule, the need to negotiate and bargain may be absent. To claim, as Lindblom does, that all policy is made incrementally is to ignore the many fundamental changes brought in by various policy-makers. We have only to think of the sweeping reforms made after the rejection of the communist regimes in eastern Europe in the 1980s to appreciate that, at certain periods in certain countries and under certain conditions, a change in policy may be sudden and radical. In the USA, the distinction between the two political parties – the Republicans and the Democrats – would appear negligible to citizens elsewhere, whose choice at election time might include parties representing various stages along the right-left ideological spectrum. Furthermore, there are examples of where the process of policy-making has proved to be closer to the model of rationality than to that of incrementalism, for example corporate planning, planning, programming and budgeting systems, and decision-making based on a cost–benefit analysis approach.

Other, Western, models of policy-making

Appreciative settings (Vickers 1965)

Policy choices are constrained by the cultural and ideological horizons of individuals and groups. Judgements of value are at the heart of the policy-making process. Conflict of interests are often deep rooted and difficult to solve. Public service organisations cannot be judged solely on the basis of customer satisfaction: there are other interests to consider. There are no built-in priorities to guide them in their multivalued choices, so they must decide what to place most value on in the concrete situation of every decision. Public services, in particular, have to be judged and their policies made by reference to multiple criteria.

Mixed scanning (Etzioni 1967)

The metaphor is of the policy-maker using two cameras: a broad-angle camera that covers a large area but not in much detail and a second camera that focuses in on those areas revealed by the first camera as requiring a more in-depth examination. The key for Etzioni is flexibility of decision-making in the light of change and uncertainty in the environment (Parsons 1995). His model is proposed as descriptive and prescriptive: the nature of some decisions is fundamental while others are incremental. Policy-makers, therefore, need to have regard to both breadth and depth depending on how they would distinguish between problems and issues requiring detailed examination and those needing a more general overview.

Planned bargaining (Challis *et al.* 1988)

Challis *et al.* (1988) have developed what they call a planning
bargaining model in which the design of a strategic framework
has to take account of the incentives and interests of all interested
parties. The model recognises the importance of rationality and
the reality of politics. In what is termed a system management
approach, the purpose is to combine and co-ordinate various
interest groups towards an agreed strategic set of policies.

Extra-rationality (Dror 1989)

One of the strongest critics of incrementalism has been Dror
(1989): he accuses incrementalism of being too conservative.
Lindblom replies that very little policy-making is revolutionary.
Drastic policy changes, he asserts, are not ordinarily possible. On
the other hand, incremental changes can be made quickly and
bring about significant policy developments in a relatively short
space of time.

Dror devised a model that includes the notion of extra-
rationality (the use of judgement, creative inventions, brainstorming, the brilliant idea that may come unexpectedly). Dror
put his model forward as a prescriptive account of how policy
ought to be made: a mix of rationality and inspiration. We might,
however, wish to distinguish between possible catalysts for
policy-making and the actual nature of the policy-making
process. In other words, a flash of inspiration may serve to insti-
gate the process. Between that moment and the evolution of the
policy statement, however, comes an often lengthy period of
development and refinement.

Summary

We need to consider whether there is much merit in developing
models of the policy-making process that attempt to provide an
ideal to aim for. These are the *prescriptive* or *normative* models.
Whatever the flaws might be in Lindblom's model, he did
attempt to combine a prescriptive and a descriptive or *explanatory* model of the policy-making process. Yet, once any commen-
tator offers a prescriptive or partly prescriptive model, we have

to ask the question, On what value system is the model based? All 'ought' statements are founded on moral principles, on a vision of an ideal world or society. Therefore, such statements are, in a sense, irrefutable unless they can be shown to be held as morally repugnant by the majority of people in society.

On the other hand, we can ask the question, To what extent are the descriptive or explanatory models derived from empirical evidence? Theories or models that emanate from particular political and cultural *milieus* cannot presume to correspond to all other political and cultural contexts. This would amount to ethno-centrism – a belief that one's own political and social system is the model on which all other systems should be based.

Thus, in academic texts, we must look for unstated assumptions about the policy-making process. We need to challenge those models presented as both prescriptive and descriptive in order to reveal how appropriate and realistic they are when viewed from another political and cultural perspective. In fact, in studying health care policies, we must be aware – on a broad scale – of who is 'managing' the key ideas, concepts and models.

Our previous discussion of power in societies helps to illuminate why various models of the policy-making process are tacit advocates of preferred political systems and power structures.

Items for discussion

1. Consider examples of health care policies that, in their construction, appear to resemble either a rational or an incremental model of the policy-making process.
2. Using the schema presented by Patton and Sawicki, examine one issue or problem in the field of health care and carry out the policy-making tasks in the order set out. Then reflect on the usefulness of this model for real-life situations.

Chapter 4 Policy implementation

Problems relating to the implementation of policy have been recognised only recently, that is, in the USA and the UK only from the 1970s onwards. There used to be a general assumption that once senior decision-makers had formulated a policy and communicated it to their own and, if appropriate, other agencies, implementation would follow almost automatically – that is, the policy or policies would be acted upon and put into effect. More recently, in the light of analysis *of* various policies, it has become increasingly recognised that having and announcing a policy is not enough to guarantee (a) that the policy will be fully implemented and (b) that it will be effective in achieving its intended objectives.

Hogwood and Gunn (1984), for example, argue that such failures have been observed in a wide range of fields, for example urban regeneration, land development, employment initiatives, the control of pollution and industrial restructuring. To this list, it is almost inevitable that we can add examples from the arena of health and health care services. Certainly, in the UK, stated policy intentions have not always been fully implemented, and the government's objectives have consequently either been thwarted or only partially successful. Harrison *et al.* (1992) have pointed out that attempts within the British NHS to shift resources towards the 'Cinderella' services for the mentally ill, mentally and physically handicapped and elderly people have not been accomplished. Similarly, the relatively recent initiative in the UK to redirect care into the community and out of hospital and other institutional settings has yet to fulfil its promise of effective support organised across professional boundaries.

The implementation gap

In certain circumstances, health care policies may only be partially implemented, may suffer delayed implementation, may not be implemented or, once put into effect, may produce completely unintended consequences. A useful framework for clarifying this concept of a 'gap' is to consider the extent to which a stated policy has achieved its stated objective or objectives. In the case of the UK care in the community initiative referred to above, all the mechanisms for putting the policy into effect were set up, legislation was passed, and health, social care and housing organisations – public, private and voluntary – started working more closely together. Yet there continue to be problems centred on the gap between intention and effect. What appears to have happened is that the whole community care enterprise is inadequately funded, and agencies 'in the field' were left by the government in power at the time to find whatever funds they could. Underlying the UK government's community care policy was a drive to reduce public expenditure on care services (Hunter 1993, Lewis and Glennerster 1996).

The above analysis is rather superficial, but it does draw attention to the fact that policy-making has to take into account, at that stage in the process, the important question of how the policy can be successfully implemented. This means that the policy process cannot be depicted visually as a neat stage-by-stage process, along the line suggested by Simon's rational model (see Chapter 3), 'implementation' being identified as a separate and later stage following on from the actual decision. The issue of implementation has to be attended to by policy-makers at the time when a possible response to a certain issue is under discussion.

The work of Pressman and Wildavsky

An influential piece of research into implementation was carried out by Pressman and Wildavsky (1973). They investigated the relative failure of the Economic Development Agency (EDA) in the city of Oakland in California, USA to achieve its key objective of providing jobs for ethnic minority groups. The EDA sought to achieve this by financial aid schemes for public works and local businesses. The results were very disappointing. A great deal of money was spent, few jobs were created yet there was no apparent participant conflict or resistance to contend with.

Pressman and Wildavsky found that the main obstacle to success was that, although the ends were agreed, the means to

41

achieving them relied on too many different agencies at central and local levels, all of which were working to different timescales. No single group had control over the total situation. In short, there was poor co-ordination.

Pressman and Wildawsky defined 'policy' as 'a hypothesis containing initial conditions and predicted consequences. If X is done at t1, then Y will result at t2'. Implementation is the process of interaction between the setting of goals and actions geared to achieving them. The conversion of the hypothesis into action these authors called a government 'programme'. Initial conditions are the passing of legislation and the securing of funds. Implementation will, they argue, become less effective as the links between all the various agencies involved in carrying out the policy form an 'implementation deficit'. The chain of command has to be capable of assembling and controlling resources, and the system able to communicate effectively and control those individuals and organisations involved in the performance of tasks (Parsons 1995). Pressman and Wildawsky later modified their original analysis towards a less 'top-down' model of the implementation process, but they initiated a flow of literature that focused on the complex nature of policy implementation.

The 'top-down' model of policy implementation

This model assumes that the process of implementation follows from decisions made at the top tier of any organisation. These decisions then have to be implemented by personnel lower down the hierarchy. Hood (1976) and Gunn (1978) adopted the thesis of Pressman and Wildawsky that stressed a quasi-military approach to ensuring that policies were implemented as intended and that, as a result, the targeted goals were attained. Hood detailed five conditions for the achievement of *perfect implementation*:

- The system in which implementation is to take place needs to resemble an army-type organisation with clear lines of authority and responsibility.
- Precise tasks and objectives are laid down.
- People carry out their specified tasks as given.
- Communication between different sections of the organisation(s) needs to be perfect.
- There are no problems created by constraints of time.

Gunn added to these items, and later, in his collaborative work with Hogwood (Hogwood and Gunn 1984), a list of eight prerequisites for perfect implementation was compiled:

1. There must be clear objectives.
2. There must be no ambiguity about the purpose of the policy.
3. Those who have to implement the policy must have the necessary commitment and skills.
4. The policy must have the support of key interest groups.
5. Sufficient time and resources are made available.
6. There are relatively few links in the implementation chain.
7. Communication between all parties is excellent.
8. There is no resistance to the policy.

These eight conditions for perfect implementation in the 'top-down' model of the policy process may be summed up under three broad headings:

1. *Change*. Has the extent of change been made clear and accepted by all interested and powerful groups affected by the policy?
2. *Control*. Can the policy-makers control the resources required in order to implement the policy and also control and, if necessary, direct all participating groups and agencies?
3. *Compliance*. Does the top level of decision-makers have complete confidence that those people who have the task of putting the policy into effect will do so without resistance?

Critiques of the top-down rational control model

This top-down prescriptive or normative model resembles the comprehensive-rational model of the policy-making process delineated by Simon, which was described in Chapter 3. It assumes that, providing the organisational mechanisms are in place and geared towards the accomplishment of clearly defined and meticulously communicated objectives, the stated policy will be fully put into effect and will, therefore, be 'successful'.

There are, it is suggested, two flaws in this model:

1. It appears to assume that human beings will tend to behave like automatons, as if we need only to set up the correct

computer program and process it by making sure that all the correct keys are pressed in the right order. Human beings, for whatever reasons, do not always behave predictably. Therefore, even if there were perfect control and compliance, there remains – at various strata within organisations – a degree of autonomy to act in ways that might not fit exactly with the policy-makers' assumptions. Lipsky (1980), as we shall see, has been influential in challenging the somewhat authoritarian rational control model of policy implementation.

2. Even if the policy has been implemented 'perfectly', the anticipated consequences may not automatically follow. What Hogwood and Gunn (1984) have described as a 'blemished theory of cause and effect' as a potential obstacle to perfect implementation is not strictly about implementation as the *process* of putting policy into operation; it has more to do with the *consequences* of a particular policy during or after the process of implementation. We return to the points made in the previous chapter about competing rationalities. In other words, the logical cause-and-effect relationship can rarely be uncontestable. Given certain, sometimes unforeseeable circumstances, a policy – even if perfectly implemented – might result in one of several possible outcomes depending on a variety of factors.

Some interesting hypothetical and actual examples of this kind of disjunction between intended and eventual policy impact illustrate the complexities involved in policy implementation.

Problems with forecasting the consequences of policy

In an article entitled, 'Laws that backfire', Bartholomew (1994) related the incident in which an aeroplane crashed in Sioux City, USA killing 111 people including a baby. The baby, like other children under the age of 2, was being carried by his parents. In the outcry that followed, politicians, parents and consumer groups demanded legislation to make baby seats compulsory. Everyone, including air crews and the airlines, agreed. Legislation was planned to implement this agreed action.

However, some academics examined other possible effects that such legislation might have. They reasoned that many couples travelling within America with their small children are relatively short of money. If they were obliged to pay for an extra seat, many would choose the cheaper alternative option of road travel. Since cars are far more likely to be involved in an accident than are aeroplanes, the likelihood of babies being killed would rise rather than fall if this policy were introduced.

This possibility of the effect being the reverse of that intended has also been noted, according to Bartholomew, by charities who provide free food to underdeveloped countries. The economic effect on local farmers has, in some cases, been negative because it annihilates their profits so that, instead of being encouraged to plant more, they are induced to plant less. In the field of social housing, the UK government of the day introduced legislation in 1967 that decontrolled rents in the privately rented sector. The intention was to stimulate a declining private sector to increase its market share. The logical argument was that, by enabling private landlords to set their own rent levels, more income would be generated, which would, in turn, be reinvested in acquiring or building new homes for rent. As it turned out, the Rent Act of 1967 led to an as yet irreversible decline in private renting as a form of housing tenure. Many landlords used the legislation to set rent at prohibitive levels so that sitting tenants who could not longer afford to remain were evicted and the houses and flats were then sold.

The 'bottom-up' model

This approach has been described as a process of consultation and negotiation that takes place between those at the 'top' and those implementing policy, and as an approach that might at times be the only means by which resistance and suspicion on the part of individuals and groups with entrenched interests might be overcome and the policy successfully implemented.

A useful contribution to recognising the influence or potential influence of lower-level 'actors' in the implementation process is that of Lipsky (1980), who coined the expression 'street level bureaucrats' to describe those people who lie at the interface between the organisation and members of the public. People such as school teachers, nurses, social workers and social security officers all play a crucial role in the kind of service that people receive. According to supporters of the bottom-up model of policy implementation, these relatively low-level personnel may have more discretion to act in the way they think appropriate than they are given credit for. Consequently, they may mediate policy imperatives in the light of competing pressures such as limited resources.

Professional and administrative practices might not actually sabotage or even undermine policy but they may certainly slow down the process of implementation. Health and social care policies, for example, that rely heavily on interprofessional collaboration might not be very effective 'on the ground' because, intentionally or unintentionally, a range of practitioners often find it difficult to work together, particularly in preplanned teams.

Baggott (1998) has remarked that joint planning between health authorities and local authorities in Britain failed to achieve a 'seamless service' in relation to implementing community care policy and legislation because of the contrasting organisational cultures and structures. As a result, certain needs were defined in different ways. For example, the majority of health authorities regarded care of the elderly mentally ill as a duty of the psychiatric services, whereas local authorities preferred to view them as clients catered for by generic services for the elderly. Compounding the problem of implementation at 'street level' are the professional rivalries between health service and local authority staff, the different planning timescales, differences in accountability and management structures, and the fact that, in many instances, the geographical jurisdictions of the two types of authority were not co-terminous.

Some potential problems in implementing health and health care policies

If we now consider some specific policies that have been put forward in order to improve the health status of nations and individuals, we can link the discussion back to the subject matter of previous sections. The statements of intent published by the WHO in a variety of documents illustrate at least two of the problems inherent in implementing policy.

First of all, the WHO definition of 'health' is so broad that the attainment of even clearly articulated objectives under this general policy 'banner' would be problematic. How, for example, could various governments agree on what constitutes 'social

well-being' among their populations? Policy as 'mission statements' cannot be successfully implemented because they are
rhetoric or 'symbolic' rather than declarations specifying explicit
and mutually agreed objectives.

Second, the policy of moving the main responsibility for
maintaining and improving the health of any nation from
government to each individual raises the question of how any
government can exercise *control* over people who do not act with
compliance. Does the government use the carrot or the stick in
order to ensure that the policy will be fully implemented and
the targets achieved?

In its strategic policy document *Affordable Health Care* (1993),
for example, the Singapore Ministry of Health stated that 'we
owe it to ourselves individually to keep fit and healthy' and that
'our health care financing is based on individual responsibility'
(p. 1). As we noted in Chapter 1, this sentiment is echoed by the
DoH in drawing up its Green Paper for England entitled *Our
Healthier Nation* (1998), although this document acknowledges
the responsibility of the government to tackle health-related
social, economic and environmental problems and widening
inequalities in health status within the population.

The document that preceded this in 1986 and its later version
in 1992, *The Health of the Nation* (DHSS 1992), was also predicated
on the *a priori* imperative of personal responsibility for maintaining a healthy lifestyle. Many of the targets set out in the 1992
document under 'Diet and Nutrition', 'Smoking' and
'HIV/AIDS' rely for their achievement on the willingness of
people to alter their habits, to become much more moderate in
their smoking and drinking, to take more exercise, to forego the
consumption of foods that contain saturated fat and, for drug
misusers, to avoid sharing injecting equipment.

The overall policy of improving the nation's health status by,
at least in part, informing people about the potential health
hazards of certain lifestyles in the hope of achieving something
approaching moral reform, brings into high relief the issue of
compliance. It also raises questions about a government's relative
commitment to those dimensions of policy-making spelt out in
Chapter 1. In order to make the attainment of certain targets a
more realistic enterprise, policies could be devised that banned
smoking, drinking alcohol and eating fatty foods with attendant
draconian penalties for people who broke the law by supplying
and consuming such products. The financial benefits that would

accrue in terms of a reduced demand upon expensive health services would clearly be offset by (a) the loss of revenue for the government through taxes on potentially health-damaging products; (b) the pragmatic concerns about the political wisdom of invoking such restrictive measures; and (c) the moral argument that – providing they do no harm to other citizens – individuals should be free to damage their own health if they so choose.

In essence, *The Health of the Nation*, as a policy document, exemplifies the inherent tension that exists between the rational control model of implementation and Lipsky's concept of street-level bureaucrats. For even though the government at that time set up a comprehensive structure of monitoring that was designed to oversee and ensure complete implementation, that is

- A ministerial Cabinet committee to co-ordinate strategy
- Three working groups
- A network of regional co-ordinators to assist with the implementation process and to disseminate information about best practice
- The establishment of focus groups for each of the key health target areas

putting appropriate mechanisms in place does not mean that the 'human factor' can be easily controlled.

This last point is clearly illustrated by comparing a policy that has the backing of legislation, and consequently the imposition of penalties for breaches of that law, and policies that mainly rely on the goodwill and compliance of staff and members of the public. Seat belt legislation and no smoking policies in the workplace and in some public areas both involve the deprivation of individual 'rights'. From time to time, police forces in many countries carry out an enforcement of the compulsory wearing of seat belts by fining drivers and/or passengers on the spot or bringing them to court, where the guilty receive a fine. In the UK, a number of public houses and bus companies have tried to impose a policy of no smoking in at least a part of the premises or vehicle. Personal experience has, however, shown that non-compliance on the part of customers has failed to invoke sufficiently punitive responses from 'street-level' staff who – in wishing to avoid conflict – more often choose to ignore behaviour that is in open defiance of the stated policy.

Another problem of implementation is that organisations – governments included – often work with different objectives at any one time. For example, a government might simultaneously be following a policy of increasing emphasis on health promotion and education with respect to the use of life-threatening drugs by young people, and a policy of stricter punitive measures against parents who are apparently not exercising proper control over their children. There will not only be issues here about what proportion of resources these two initiatives should be granted in relation to each other, but also the question of how the government can identify the extent to which each policy is or is not helping to reduce the incidence of drug use among young people. This is related to the area of policy evaluation, which we shall deal with in the next chapter.

Even when policies appear to be fully implemented on a continuing basis, the intended result may not happen. Hogwood and Gunn (1986) would call this the problem of a blemished cause-and-effect theory. That is to say, the underlying logic 'If we do X, then Y will follow' is flawed in some way. As we have noted earlier, a policy will sometimes turn out to have an effect opposite to that intended, even though it has been properly implemented. In many cases, the reason for such an unexpected outcome is the human factor. An example to add to those already given is that the provision of health care services free at the point of need would arguably so enhance the general health status of a population that the demand for such services would decrease over time; a healthier population would make fewer demands for services, and gradually the funding of these services would decrease. Yet we know that this logic – although not unreasonable in theory – has proved wrong in many countries: the provision of services has served only to stimulate demand.

Summary

Top-down and bottom-up models of policy implementation are not, in themselves, completely adequate facsimiles of how policy is put into practice. As Elmore (1978) has stated, no single model captures the full complexity of the implementation process.

A quotation from a book written by Walt (1994) aptly sums up the main issues concerning implementation as part of the policy-making process:

> implementation cannot be seen as part of a linear or sequential process, in which political dialogue takes place at the policy formulation stage, and implementation is undertaken by administrators or managers. It is a complex, interactive process, in which implementers themselves may affect the way policy is executed, and are active in formulating change and innovation. (p. 177)

The provision of services free at the point of need has indeed considerably helped to reduce the risks and prevalence of many diseases. It has greatly contributed in many countries to extending life expectancy and reducing the infant mortality rate. Yet the system has been a victim of its own success. People's expectations of health standards have increased, and – as we shall note in subsequent chapters dealing with health care planning – the demand for expensive health care interventions seems to be insatiable.

Items for discussion

> 1. With reference to any aspect of health care services, consider the reasons – hypothetical or actual – why a policy does not appear to have achieved its objectives.
> 2. Discuss the relevance of the concept of street-level bureaucrat to any health care setting with which you are familiar.

Chapter 5   Policy Evaluation

Governments and health care agencies use a variety of methods to check whether their 'performance' meets certain standards. This concern with such matters as 'quality control' is a recent phenomenon in the history of the health care services. In the field of education, however, there has been, in several countries, a series of formal evaluations designed to assess the impact of innovative teaching/learning programmes on particular sets of students (Cronbach 1963, 1982, Mathison 1992).

The term *formal evaluation* is the one that applies to the main contents of this chapter. This differs from various other methods of attempting to measure performance, which are dealt with more extensively by Phillips *et al.* (1994). Formal evaluation is a form of social science research that often attempts to discover whether a specified form or programme of interventions has achieved its objective(s). A useful framework to apply to the process of formal evaluation is the system model, in which an organisation's activities may be characterised as a quasi-production process involving the linked components:

- *Inputs*: for example funding, staff and values
- *Process*: the manner in which services are provided, including procedures, communication and, generally, the nature of interaction between people
- *Outputs*: the goods and services provided
- *Outcomes*: the impact of inputs, process and outputs on key stake-holders involved in the health care system.

This last-named item – outcomes – has come to be a dominant concern within health care organisations and for governments in many countries, and we will devote part of Chapter 8 to the issue of health care outcomes.

Key components of a system model

One advantage of the system model is that it acts as a reminder that health care policy-makers and implementers might accord different emphases to certain aspects of health care systems and organisational objectives. Medical practitioners, for example, are likely to focus on achieving clinical efficacy as the primary criterion for assessing policy as it adds to or detracts from the achievement of high-quality treatment for patients and their own professional satisfaction. On the other hand, managers of hospitals and commissioning agencies are likely to assess policies by reference to quantifiable targets, such as patient throughput or the reduction of waiting lists, as well as those measures relating to the comparative cost-effectiveness of various forms of medical intervention.

The generic yardstick of *efficiency* – the relationship between inputs and outputs – is also a criterion that governments would apply in order to evaluate the 'success' of policies involving the allocation of public funds to health care service provision.

In contrast, patients may well place greater stress on the need for policies that aim to maintain and improve upon the *process* of care, the quality of human interaction between health care practitioners, administrators and other health care staff and the individual patient. Health care policies often have to be framed along lines that attempt to achieve a number of different objectives affecting a variety of stake-holders. Referring back to Chapters 1 and 4, compromises usually have to be made in making sure that policies take into account economic, moral and ideological concerns and that these are sufficiently balanced in eventual policies in order to minimise the risk of non-compliance and electoral repercussions. Within the UK context, for example, the need for policy evaluation was declared very clearly in a government document (DoE 1992) stating that all Cabinet papers proposing new policies:

> should state clearly what is to be achieved, by whom, at what cost and how the policies are to be measured and evaluated... Evaluation is a key management tool... It is also the means by which value for money is assessed, and for reviewing the effects of a policy either in operation or after it has been completed. (p. 3)

Evaluation: the rationale

The above emphasis on the management perspective and on 'value for money' as a virtual synonym for 'cost-effectiveness' tends to limit the purpose of formal, systematic evaluation. The need for the evaluation of health care services may be argued in the following terms:

1. The sharper focus on user and carer in the planning and design of care programmes logically demands a rational assessment of whether the services adequately match expectation.
2. The shift in many countries from traditional modes of residential and institutional care in the community is based on certain premises relating to appropriateness, equity, choice and effectiveness. These criteria are, by themselves, little more than expressions of faith. Health and social care in action have to be judged as accurately as possible using these criteria, and perhaps others, as the starting point for the process of formal evaluation.
3. The very process of evaluation affords an opportunity for user participation in decision-making. By involving users in the initial stages of selecting what should be evaluated and according to what criteria, the assumptions that may be harboured by professional people about what constitutes an effective process, content and outcome of interventions can be tested against service users' views on these essential issues.
4. 'Policy as programme' evaluation should also help to clarify questions about prioritising and allocating resources more efficiently and more cost-effectively within designated service areas, both within and across agencies.
5. Particularly with regard to innovative schemes involving vulnerable people, monitoring and evaluation, and the dissemination of findings, can inform others about examples of best practice.
6. Published material derived from sound empirical research can lay the foundation for a body of knowledge informing policy-makers about the relationship between inputs, processes, outputs and outcomes.

In addition, we can list below, almost at random, a number of questions relating to a variety of largely unexplored issues central to such key concepts as *quality of service, professionalism, consumerism* and *cost-effectiveness*:

- How do professionals know that they are doing a good job?
- Do they need to know, and if so, for what reasons?
- How do we know whether the professional's and the manager's idea of a 'good' policy matches that of other interested parties?
- What do different stake-holders mean by a 'successful' treatment?
- How can we evaluate the process of nursing care?
- How can a funding agency or primary care group know whether it is getting value for money?
- How do we know whether a particular care programme or form of intervention is 'better' than any other?

The impact of evaluation research on policy-making

As Walt (1994) has pointed out, there are two differing sets of opinions about the influence of evaluation and other types of research finding upon policy-makers. Looking at health services research, Harrison *et al.* (1992) concluded :

In the United States, as in the UK, the relationship between research findings, however conclusive, and organisational and policy change is a tenuous one. There is certainly no automatic translation of research into policy. (p. 168)

A more optimistic point of view is that new information derived from research filters through into the political arena, where major decisions are made and become part of the policy-makers' thinking in a *diffused* rather than a *specific* way. Evaluation raises new questions, is 'illuminative' (Hamilton *et al.* 1977) rather than explanatory, and has a cumulative effect rather than an immediate and direct influence on public policy.

Yet we can identify cases in which formal evaluation has contributed directly to the creation of policy. In the UK, for example, the extensive pilot studies carried out at the University of Kent into the costs and effectiveness of intensive domiciliary care services for elderly people undoubtedly influenced the government in its commitment to a new direction away from hospital and residential care to care in the community for vulnerable, elderly people and for ex-mental health patients and patients with learning difficulties.

Politics and evaluation

Whether the results of formal evaluation contribute in one way or another to health care policy will depend to a large extent on whether the data produced are compatible with the ideology, aspirations and resource commitments of those who have the power to decide. Surveys carried out in the UK have identified a close correlation between health status and socio-economic factors such as unemployment, housing and income. The Black Report (DHSS 1980), for example, produced evidence that people who were relatively disadvantaged materially were statistically more likely to suffer from bad physical and mental health. Certain geographical areas where these problems were particularly severe were identified. The logical policy flowing from this data would have been to prioritise those areas for government spending on health promotion and intervention programmes as a form of positive discrimination.

However, the government that commissioned the report had been voted out of office by the time the report was published, and the incoming government held no ideological commitment to a policy of increased, or even redistribution of, public expenditure. As a consequence, the findings of the report were never acted upon. With a Labour government returned to power in 1997, their White Paper *Our Healthier Nation* (DoH 1998) takes as its first principle the need to reduce inequalities in health status among the population of England. This is the reality that evaluators must face. Policy-making is a political activity that does not have to yield to the logic of apparent 'facts'. In this sense, 'reality' is what those in power choose to define as 'reality'. We will return to the notion of policy-making as the *rationalisation of values*. Whose values prevail will depend not so much on the validity of formal evaluation research findings as on the recognition by policy-makers of the validity of claims for action (or inaction) by certain stake-holders.

Stake-holders and their values

In the planning and delivery of any public service, there is always a wide range of stake-holders, including those who are paying for the services, those who are intended to benefit from the services, the front-line professionals who provide the services and the managers who plan and co-ordinate the services. In some respects, all the stake-holders want the services to be successful, but there are likely to be marked differences in opinion about what constitutes 'success'. (Smith and Cantley 1985)

Those who pay directly or indirectly might, for example, be a government on behalf of its citizens, or the intended beneficiary who may be expected to pay for health care services through an intermediary such as an insurance company, through a government-controlled savings scheme or directly at the point of service. In the UK, this category would also include GP fundholders and district health authorities (DHAs). Those who pay are the service customers, and they are likely to emphasise value for money in their expectations of the service in question. The aspects of value for money likely to be considered particularly important will be *economy* and *efficiency*, especially elements of those that relate to the level of expenditure (Thomas and Palfrey 1996). Purchasers might also be interested in *equity* because DHAs and social services departments are charged with the task of identifying and assessing health and social care needs in their areas and then purchasing services to meet those needs.

Intended beneficiaries

It could be argued that every individual or group involved at any time with health care services, be it a government, purchasers, all personnel working in the service, the public at large or individual patients and their families, is an intended beneficiary. Here, we shall focus on the individual. In this case, the most relevant evaluative criteria are likely to be:

- *Accessibility*, in terms of location, waiting times and affordability
- *Appropriateness*: the relevance to the patient's perceived needs

- *Responsiveness*, which relates to the manner in which the person's concerns, desires and general well-being are treated by staff.

Some people might also wish to exercise *choice* about which doctor or which hospital should provide the service.

Professionals, managers and politicians

Professionals

Medical practitioners, nurses and para-medical staff will derive a sense of achievement if they are allowed the autonomy to decide the kind of help a particular patient needs and the best way of providing that help. Such autonomy is likely to lead to the professional feeling a sense of responsibility for the outcomes of intervention (Hackman and Oldham 1980). In this context, criteria such as *effectiveness* and *appropriateness* will be emphasised.

Managers

On the other hand, managers will probably be most concerned with *efficiency* and *accountability*. They will need to justify their performance in terms of *cost-effectiveness* and also to ensure that their decisions are congruent with those of the professionals whose work they are there to facilitate and monitor.

Politicians

Politicians will also have keen regard to the criterion of *accountability* – to their colleagues, their constituents, their party and the general public. In these days, when health targets are being set at a global level and many of the more developed countries are acting as donors to assist less-developed countries to provide public health and health care services, accountability can also apply between nations.

Government ideology will largely determine the emphasis laid on other criteria. For example, the objective of achieving *social equity* in the distribution of resources and the levels of health experienced by the population reflects a commitment rooted in a value system that accepts good health as a human right rather than a desirable commodity to be bought in the marketplace. Where governments subsidise health care provision, they will clearly want to be assured that they are receiving value for money as defined by the relationship between costs and outputs (efficiency) and between costs and outcomes (cost-effectiveness or cost-utility).

Criteria for evaluating the quality of health care services

A useful starting point for classifying criteria for evaluating services has been suggested by Maxwell (1984) in relation to the quality of services. His suggested criteria are:

- Effectiveness
- Efficiency
- Equity
- Acceptability
- Accessibility
- Appropriateness (relevance to need).

Effectiveness

Effectiveness can be defined as the achievement of stated objectives. The use of this yardstick for evaluating performance depends on the specification of explicit and clear objectives. As we shall note later in this chapter in discussing the work of Smith and Cantley (1985), clarifying unambiguous objectives may be highly problematic. If appropriate, objectives can be measured by quantifiable indicators such as the response times in answering telephone calls and other means of communication, the through-put of patients in hospital and waiting times for operations. In the context of clinical care, a similar concept – efficacy – is applied. A drug or medical treatment such as an operation is efficacious if it appears to have achieved its objective of, for example, the relief of pain or the cure of disease.

Being effective is not, however, to be equated in every case with providing a good-quality service. If objectives are inappropriate, effectiveness will not mean much. For example, targets that are too easy to achieve or that serve morally questionable purposes will fall into this category. Effectiveness in itself might also have little regard for the costs involved. Like other criteria for evaluating health care, it has a limited scope for providing information about performance.

Efficiency

Efficiency as the ratio of benefits (in terms of either outputs or outcomes) to costs can be increased in the following ways:

- Increasing benefits while not increasing costs
- Reducing costs but not reducing benefits
- Increasing benefits and costs but increasing the former more than the latter
- Reducing costs while increasing benefits (the ultimate in efficiency).

One of the difficulties of using efficiency as an evaluation criterion is that costs and benefits can be very difficult to measure accurately. On the face of it, costs would seem to be highly amenable to calculation provided that accounting procedures are sufficiently detailed, meticulous and capable of generating easily accessible data. The economist's notion of costs, however, is rather complex and includes, as one example, the idea of *opportunity costs*, which are measures of what is being given up in order to use resources in health care. Allocating money within any health care system relies on choices having to be made between alternatives: between different medical treatments, for example, or between different types of intervention – invasive or less invasive surgery. In a series of articles, Robinson (1993 a–e) deals with all the main forms of economic evaluation.

Benefits are difficult to assess both in principle and in practice because they usually entail an analysis of intangibles such as *quality of life*. Cost utility analysis – as we shall note in Chapter 9 in the Oregon approach to prioritising health care spending – uses this problematic concept as an integral component of an allocative formula.

Equity

One useful way to conceptualise this abstract term is to regard it as a move towards treating equally people with equal needs. This alludes to a process that is seen to be fair. For example, people placed on a waiting list for a hip replacement operation might regard as equitable a system that constructed the list in chronological order on a first-come, first-served basis. Conversely, treating people differently according to their different needs is also essential to the concept of equity. The original meaning of *triage* was the selection, in times of war or catastrophe, for treatment of those casualties most likely to survive. The term is frequently applied in accident and emergency units in hospitals where selection for treatment is based on the criterion of urgent attention being given to patients with the most serious injuries – almost the opposite of the original meaning.

Acceptability

One application of this criterion is in the context of standards of services. Of course, in relation to the previous criterion – equity – an unjust system for allocating resources would also be unacceptable. The problem lies in identifying a consensus about what is deemed to be inequitable or unfair. It is highly improbable that any country would adopt a completely *laissez-faire* strategy for health care since the capacity to pay directly for all services would seriously disadvantage those people with relatively little purchasing power, and this would contravene most people's moral sensitivities. Inordinately lengthy waiting times for treatment, the neglect of vulnerable people, and unhygienic environments are all examples of health-related standards that fall well below an acceptable level.

Accessibility

This term can be interpreted in a number of ways. Any health care policy that discriminates in any way so that certain patients have priority over others is, in effect, announcing that the accessibility of services will differ between people in need of help. This is essentially the reasoning behind policies that accept prioritising as an inevitable feature of health care administration. Accessibility to health care services will also be discriminatory wherever private facilities exist since this option is not available for everyone in the community. Some potential patients will be able to receive treatment at primary, secondary or tertiary levels, while others who are unable to afford to pay for private health insurance or to pay a fee for private health care will have to wait.

Accessibility can also be expressed as the physical means of receiving health care. The ambulance services are organised in order to enhance the accessibility of hospital treatment; GP practices and primary health care clinics might organise a rota for out-of-hours services, including home visits; ramps are constructed for disabled persons to gain easier access to buildings. In Maxwell's (1984) catalogue, accessibility is a key attribute of a good-quality health service, but policies and practices that debar sections of the population can lead to services that are of high quality in clinical terms even though access to them is limited. There are numerous examples of high-quality products and services that are not accessible to everyone.

Appropriateness

From all stake-holders' points of view, appropriateness would seem to be an important criterion for evaluating health care policies as they affect the provision and delivery of services. Of course, appropriateness is capable of being interpreted from several perspectives: value for money, clinical expertise, professional judgement or consumer preference. Whereas acceptability often relates to standards of services, it does not necessarily mean that a service that is of a high standard will be appropriate in terms of either cost or individual choice. Several recipients of domiciliary care during the period of a pilot community care project were asked by the research team attached to the project whether the home care services that they were receiving were of an acceptable standard. A number of these elderly people felt that the service was first class. However, when they were asked which form of help they would list as their number one priority, many of them chose help or care that was different from what they were receiving (Phillips *et al.* 1994).

Other criteria for evaluation

Following on from the work of Le Grand and Robinson (1994), four additional criteria could be added:

- Accountability
- Ethical considerations
- Responsiveness
- Choice.

These, in total, ten criteria are probably those which would adequately cover the various yardsticks applied by the range of health services stake-holders. Others could also be considered.

Equality can be considered as part of the criterion of equity, that is, equal treatment for people with equal needs. Its application could also lead to charges of unfairness if, for example, no provisions were made for people on a low income to be charged less than more affluent patients for prescriptions.

Economy is rather a limited criterion since it focuses exclusively on how costs can be reduced or maintained at current levels.

Quality of life is such a disputed concept that there is little guarantee that different people would define it in similar terms.

The above criteria, and others referred to earlier in this chapter, present a menu from which to select according to the nature of what is being evaluated and who influences the actual design of the evaluation. On this last point, it is extremely unlikely that all stake-holders will agree on the criteria to be used in a formal evaluation and on how the criteria are to be weighted. Those supported by the most powerful group(s) are most likely to be adopted. In the realm of health care services, however, the system model component of 'outcomes' is no longer defined merely in terms of clinical 'success'. Different criteria from the patient's perspective are also considered to be relevant in helping to clarify what is meant by a 'successful' treatment; these include the acceptability of certain possible side-effects, and long-term versus short-term physical and/or mental conditions. We shall return to this particular topic of health care outcomes in Chapter 9.

Who should carry out an evaluation?

It is implicit in many texts on evaluation that the expert outsider will be the most appropriate person to carry out the evaluation. This will normally be a trained academic or consultant. The advantages of employing such a person are seen to be these:

- Someone outside the organisation is more likely to be objective and, therefore, avoid biased conclusions.
- The evaluation findings are more likely to be taken seriously by the commissioning agency because they have been produced by an expert.
- Key participants are more likely to co-operate with someone who is not part of their own organisation.

These are all valid points, but they do not in themselves amount to a sufficient cause for appointing an expert outsider to conduct the evaluation. In some situations, people might co-operate more sincerely and openly with a person similar in age, gender and social background to themselves. The point is that who carries out the evaluation should only be decided after the purpose and design of the evaluation has been determined. The argument in favour of the 'expert' evaluator stems from the traditional idea that social science research should correspond closely to the techniques of the natural sciences. The expert outsider then plays the role of the neutral scientist who meticulously observes, records and, ultimately, passes judgement.

However, *ethnographic* approaches to evaluation place an emphasis more on participatory and action research in which participants are no longer the *objects* of the research but become co-researchers. The design of such evaluations will feature *formative evaluation* in which there is a continuous feedback and review of progress.

Pluralistic evaluation

The need to take into consideration the views of several stakeholders in evaluating successful performance in the health care sector demands an approach to formal evaluation that goes beyond a single yardstick of 'success'. To conclude, for example, that a hospital is providing a first-class service to the public merely because patients are processed efficiently in terms of throughput, for example bed usage and occupation/vacancy rates, or in terms of waiting times in outpatient clinics, would be to distort the picture. There are many dimensions to any organisation's activities. An innovative programme could prove efficient in managerial and administrative terms but be a relative disaster as far as staff morale was concerned.

For this reason, Smith and Cantley (1985) and Palfrey *et al.* (1992) have advocated a pluralistic approach to evaluation. This involves the inclusion of all major stake-holders in the design of the evaluation research and in its process; it also involves the application of more than one method of data collection in order to 'cross-check' the data generated. The advantage of employing this type of evaluation methodology is that it is more sensitive to the varying interpretations of 'success' or 'good quality' than are more limited devices. It shows, for example, that policies, programmes and processes can be successful in some aspects and defective in others. By using different participants' definitions of the situation, pluralistic evaluation gathers data on the criteria used by different individuals and groups in recognising the achievement of objectives and in the appropriateness, for them, of those objectives.

Evaluation research designs

The view expressed by Smith and Cantley (1985) is that many formal evaluations are built upon questionable assumptions:

● The presumption of rationality
● The presumption of the experimentalist ideal
● The presumption of consensus.

In brief, their critique of traditional evaluation up to the middle 1980s of health care policies and programmes runs along the following lines:

First, the rationalist model of the policy process is (as we noted in Chapter 3) an ideal model. In practice, policy-making is often confused, and evaluations must reflect that. In addition, the rational model deals with clear goals whereas ambiguity and confusion of purpose are not at all unusual features of organisations. Objectives vary across different groups. Goals of services are complex, multiple and often conflicting, varying over time and between contexts. Also, in many services, valid output measures are not available and need to be investigated and clarified before the evaluation process can begin.

The second presumption that is frequently made in evaluative research is the desirability of experimental or quasi-experimental research designs such as the randomised controlled trial advocated by Cochrane (1972). These test various interventions against alternatives and use experimental and control groups. In laboratory conditions in which drugs are tested, such an approach has obvious merits. However, in the world that involves the complexities of human interaction, Smith and Cantley – drawing upon a body of literature that challenges the appropriateness of an experimental design for evaluations – maintain that the difficulties in controlling external variables, the ethical issues involved in assigning people to experimental and control groups, the ability to test only two alternative programmes and the potential bias exerted by individuals who may be aware of the experiment – all inhibit the validity of any findings resulting from the evaluation.

Third, people who work within or who have contact with an organisation do not necessarily share the same view about what ought to be the dominant goals of the organisation. Different interested parties might attach differing values to particular areas of activity. The presumption of consensus is likely to reflect the values attached to selective organisational goals according to management perspectives.

Pluralistic evaluation places a value on a range of interpretations about the quality of standards and attempts to replace a positivist paradigm of investigation, that is that there is a reality 'out there' waiting to be discovered, with a subjectivist or phenomenological paradigm in which the evaluator is interested in how various stake-holders construct their *own* realities.

Summary

Formal evaluation, done properly, is rarely a cheap endeavour. In order to gain access to highly 'rich' data, evaluators sometimes have to spend considerable time gaining the confidence of all interested parties, even when those carrying out the evaluation are part of the programme. There may on occasions be tension between the research commissioners and those carrying out the evaluation. A longitudinal evaluation lasting for a year or more may promise to produce more convincing conclusions than research of a shorter timescale, but this may well lead to difficulties in finally assessing whether a specific programme or other external factors have influenced outcomes.

We need, perhaps, to learn to accept that the result of formal evaluation may be highly contextual in terms of place and time, and that the impact of one set of services for certain people with similar needs may not be the same in another place at another time. Nevertheless, formal evaluation has an important part to play among the range of mechanisms designed to make the providers of health care services more accountable to the general public.

Items for discussion

> 1. From the point of view of managers, clinical staff and patients, what would be the main attributes of a 'good quality' out-patient service?
> 2. How can we attempt to distinguish between quality of *service* and quality of *life*?

Chapter 6 Health care planning

Lee and Mills (1985) have characterised planning as 'the process of deciding how the future should be different from the present, what changes are necessary and how these changes should be brought about'. Could this not, however, also be a close definition of 'policy-making?' Perhaps it differs in two aspects:

1. *Planning* assumes change, whereas policy – as we have noted in Chapter 1 – might confirm the need for no change, being merely a reaffirmation of the *status quo*.
2. *Planning* is concerned with the 'how', that is, it is focused on the means by which change can be brought about, including the details of policy implementation.

The difference can, perhaps, be more clearly illustrated by an example. A health authority might refer to its '5-Year Plan' but not to its '5-Year Policy'.

The 'Plan' sets out a timescale for the implementation of a key policy or set of polices. The purpose of planning systems is to provide a means by which policies will be translated into action. Planning also assumes that a calculated intervention will improve the future and that future events can be, in some part, predicted.

As highlighted above, planning has been defined as:

the process of deciding how the future should be different from the present, what changes are necessary and how these changes should be brought about. (Lee and Mills 1985, p. 30)

This definition assumes that change *will* be necessary whereas, in the short term, policy-makers might be content to maintain the *status quo*. Planning takes place within a policy context. It may be described as a 'structured programme of implementation within a framework of stated policy', although the very act of trying to anticipate future demands for health care services might initiate policy. Planning is the mechanism by which strategy targets are actioned and finance is committed to the achievement of strategic objectives.

'Health planning' is different from 'health care planning' because health planning may identify measures – such as improved highways, safer cars, a cleaner environment and work safety measures – that need to be taken other than through health care as a public sector responsibility. As we noted in Chapter 1, we concentrate in this book on the more restricted area of health care planning.

The purposes of planning

To improve decision-making and manage resources more efficiently and more effectively

In developing countries, finance and skilled manpower are usually extremely scarce. In more developed countries, concern for the scarcity of resources stems from the continual growth of high-cost, capital-intensive and mostly hospital-based medical care.

To counteract territorial inequities

In both developed and developing countries, there is often an identified imbalance between the resources allocated to different regions. Some, for example rural as opposed to urban, areas may suffer from relatively poor health status compared with the rest of the country and may also have worse access to medical care.

To clarify priorities for health care expenditure

This could involve decisions concerning:

- The merits of different types of health care interventions: should resources be concentrated more on primary care and health education?
- On different patient groups: elderly or infants, maternity cases or schoolchildren
- On different clinical groups, for example, cancer patients or cases of acute rather than chronic conditions

- Different categories of health care expenditure, such as clinical research, nurse recruitment, high technology equipment or health promotion or community care.

To encourage the provision of an effective database for decision-making

Planning demands information that is up to date, accurate and comprehensive. Some of this, such as morbidity and mortality data will be gathered on a national scale. Epidemiological data can also be generated and analysed in order to identify trends at regional, area and more local levels. Hospital and GP records can contribute to health care planning in terms of the development of specialties in response to the incidence of certain diseases and in terms of strategies for health promotion campaigns.

To put policy into staged operation

In many cases, a policy as programme cannot be implemented in full on a prearranged date. Much legislation makes provision for the phasing-in of specific legislative measures over a period of time. For example, in the UK, the NHS and Community Care Act of 1990 was not fully operational until 1993. The reasons for staged implementation may relate to the following:

1. There may be a need to put into place important structural and organisational changes. For example, it would be premature to devolve responsibilities and budgets to lower levels of management unless appropriately trained staff were in post in order to cope with such change.
2. Funds might not be available to put a policy into effect. A decision to close hospitals and discharge former mental health patients or persons with learning disabilities, for example, ought not to be implemented overnight without adequate resources being made available to support such vulnerable people in the community.
3. A health care policy, such as the development of more competition to provide health care services and a clearer emphasis on consumer choice, might need to be tested out in one

geographical or service area in order to check its effectiveness in reducing the extent of government intervention in the health care system and/or to gauge public opinion about the new policy in action.

To measure performance

As point 3 above suggests, planning is a process that can incorporate a monitoring function. At macro (central government) and micro (for example hospital/clinic) levels, policy can be reviewed if its objectives have been clearly defined and the criteria for evaluating performance have been articulated. 'Performance' might, therefore, refer to enhancing the cost-effectiveness of some aspects of a health care system, to effectiveness in reducing waiting lists for hospital treatment, or to the efficacy of a specific health care intervention.

Resources and demands

Planning is a future-orientated activity, central to whose purpose is the judicious use of resources, not least within the province of health care, because publicly funded or part-funded health care systems have to provide accessible services that give value for money. Governments are accountable not only to the public, but also to a system of auditing that scrutinises the ways in which funds are used.

Although, as we shall see in Chapter 9, there are dissident voices who would contest such a claim, economists and most politicians would agree that, as far as health care is concerned, there is infinite demand but only finite resources available in order to try to cope with that demand. Strategies, therefore, have to be adopted that will attempt to deal with this imperfect market. Far from diminishing the need for the public to use health care services, more and more sophisticated clinical and therapeutic measures to combat disease and impairment seem to have the effect of increasing the demand for health care services. An ever-increasing supply can, instead of staunching demand, serve to heighten people's expectations, which in turn leads to more demands being made on suppliers.

There are various strategies that can be adopted in attempting to maintain a reasonable balance between resources and demands within a health care context, as described below.

Suppress the demand and control supply

In countries that operate a heavily subsidised health care service, the introduction of fees at the point of service can serve to make people think twice about whether they really need treatment or a consultation about their health. The withdrawal of facilities – the closure of hospital wards, of specialty provision or of the hospital itself – could reduce the demand for tertiary (specialist facilities) or secondary (general hospital) care and redirect the demand for less costly primary care.

Controlling or suppressing demand or supply is sometimes referred to as 'de-marketing'. Mark and Brennan (1995) refer to evidence from 12 European countries showing that health care costs can be most easily contained by regulating supply and consequently demand. This is certainly what the government in Singapore had in mind when it set out its policy to 'regulate the overall number of doctors and specialists' and 'control the total number of hospital beds'. (Singapore Ministry of Health 1993, p. 25)

Stimulate demand

Following on from the last point, many countries rely more and more on health promotion and health education campaigns and services in order to try to avoid the onset of preventable diseases. Efforts are made to encourage people to adopt healthier lifestyles, to attend screening programmes and to have regular medical check-ups. Money is spent on advertising the benefits of such preventive measures in the hope that considerably more money will be saved in the longer term by delaying patients' admission to comparatively costly hospital treatments. In some instances, a government will bring in laws not only to safeguard its citizens, but also to save money. The compulsory wearing of seat-belts and, in many countries, the legal requirement for vehicles to pass a roadworthiness test are examples of where 'demand' for preventive measures is 'stimulated' by the threat of financial penalties.

Setting priorities and rationing

Rationing is, in a sense, a negative concept; it involves setting stricter budgets and is a way of restricting the supply of goods or services to individuals. It usually applies to everyone, for example in times of economic hardship, when each person is allowed only a specified amount of certain types of food. Dieting is a form of self-rationing. In the context of health care, putting people on a waiting list for treatment has been described as the main example of 'implicit rationing'. Because distinctions are drawn between individual cases, however, this gate-keeping function has more to do with prioritising the more 'deserving' cases according to the clinical judgements of medical practitioners.

Setting priorities – prioritising – has a more positive aspect. Working still within defined budgets, decisions are made about where resources should be allocated on the basis of an agreed scheme. This practice is inescapably rooted in value judgements about where and how the greatest *benefits* are likely to be gained in response to identified need. Planning health care services ultimately involves choices, as we shall reiterate below. Unless health care is regarded as a commodity good – the USA probably coming closest to this interpretation of medical intervention – that has to be paid for like any other product or service in the marketplace, governments will make provision for some form of subsidised health care. Yet, because of increasing demand, some limits may have to be imposed upon the range of treatments offered. Attempts to attach values to various health care services and treatments, and thus to prioritise them, have been gaining ground. Some examples will be dealt with later in this chapter.

Forecasting future demand

Drawing upon data generated through epidemiological research, health trends, demographic data and service utilisation, forecasts can be made about future needs and demands for services. While long-term 'crystal ball' scenarios can be very useful in focusing the mind of politicians, professionals and administrators on the probable impact of such developments as technological innovations, drugs research and the re-emergence of diseases, most planning decisions concentrate more on how best to make existing policies work than on responding to as yet unverified assumptions.

Key issues in health care planning

Planning is – as Lee and Mills (1985) point out – to do with making *choices*, choices to be made within a policy framework. One broad strategic policy, for example, might be to develop health care services in the community, based perhaps on clinics and/or domiciliary services. Within this policy framework, choices have to be made about the allocation of resources. Should funding be increased by X per cent for ex-mental health patients or by Y per cent for people with learning difficulties?

Choices also have to be made concerning decisions taken with a certain 'time-horizon', that is, short term or long term. Such decisions will be conditioned by political concerns about the probability of any planned changes producing beneficial results within the lifetime of a particular government, 'beneficial' not just for citizens, but also, of course, for the government in power.

The dominant issue is perhaps the way in which some equation is reached between demand and resources. How can resources be used in order to achieve maximum health gain? Should members of the public as well as politicians, managers and professionals be involved in this realm of decision-making? On which and on whose sets of values should planning be based? In summary, planning is an exercise in *control* – over resources, over demand, perhaps even over professionals.

Factors affecting planning

As we discussed in Chapter 4 on 'implementation', external circumstances beyond the control of policy-makers sometimes alter the course of events, with the result that the intended consequences of policy are not realised. No policy analyst, politician or expert adviser can forecast the future with certainty, but the probability of things going wrong can be reduced. One way of doing this is to test out a policy initiative in a pilot scheme and to evaluate its results. Other contingencies, however, are not predictable.

Political stability

In some countries, a change of government may herald so drastic a revision or reversal of health policies that plans will have to be rewritten. Frequent government changes or a high degree of political instability may undermine the capacity to make secure, long-term plans.

Economic stability

Planners in the public sector need to feel some assurance that public expenditure projections in general – and those for the health budget in particular – are reliable. Planning has to be sufficiently robust (for example, by using a range of resource assumptions to formulate alternative scenarios) to withstand high levels of inflation, a sudden escalation in capital or drug costs, or changes in resource availability.

Co-operation

For planning decisions to be translated into action, it is necessary for decision-makers to satisfy themselves that those agencies, organisations and groups of people responsible for action are committed to ensuring that the plans do in fact reach fruition. Policy-makers sometimes need to set up formal arrangements in order to monitor progress at decentralised points in the implementation structure. The role of management in hospitals, for example, could be paramount in trying to ensure that strategic plans involving patient throughput, an investment in new technology, and prioritising according to agreed criteria and formulae become reality.

Technical infrastructure

Planning will have little chance of success unless appropriate methodologies and techniques are available to produce relevant and accurate information, unless competent personnel in the relevant specialties and disciplines are employed in adequate numbers, and unless there is an organisational structure appropriately designed to sustain and promote the planning activity.

Origins and development of health care planning

Planning within health care systems has been adopted from corporate planning in commercial companies. Faced with the problems of organisational size and complexity, and with sensitivity to technological change, many organisations set out to improve the co-ordination between departments and divisions, to manage growth in a structured and efficient manner, to develop sound investment policy and to put into place sound mechanisms for anticipating technological change.

Corporate planning in the UK and USA developed in the 1950s and 60s and was to bring the following benefits:

- It forced management to think systematically about the future.
- It created a sense of collective direction.
- It provided criteria for assessing proposals for expansion and contraction.
- It provided a basis for resource planning (especially finance and staffing).

From the mid-1960s the WHO began to transfer planning ideas from the private, commercial world to the health sector. Local government in the UK also realised the virtue of corporate planning so that different spending departments and committees were aware of each other's plans and commitments. Heads of department met together regularly as a senior executive in order to co-ordinate activities and gain an overall picture of the present and potential futures.

In the 1970s, the Department of Health and Social Security (DHSS) in the UK set out the main objectives to be achieved by a comprehensive planning system based on accurate and continually updated information. Planning was intended (DHSS 1976) to:

- Improve decision-making and manage resources better
- Enhance cost-effectiveness by means of a coherent pattern of services
- Provide an objective, factual information base for decision-making
- Enhance communication with local decision makers
- Ensure a more rational use of resources
- Produce corporate and comprehensive plans
- Help to reduce inequalities in health care.

Future studies

One influential method of forecasting future health care demands and the means to cope with the need for health care services is that of 'future studies'. This approach attempts to take the future as the baseline and look backward to the present. It reveals alternatives and the probability of their happening and, in this way, provides a context for policy and planning decisions.

In particular, future studies take into account the rapid development of new technologies, not only in medical care, treatment and diagnosis, but also in the broad area of information technology and computer applications. Analysis is made of the potential impact of such developments on resource allocation and prioritising, on the location of health and social care, for example day hospitals or people's own homes rather than conventional hospitals, and on staffing implications. There will be more coverage and critique of these types of studies in Chapter 7.

The Oregon plan

Probably the most ambitious attempt at setting health care priorities was undertaken in the state of Oregon in the USA. Other countries have studied the Oregon plan and are carrying out similar exercises involving the public in health care planning. A detailed description of the plan is contained in the book by Coast *et al.* (1996). We shall, therefore, give only a brief summary of the origins of this innovative approach to planning and set out some commentators' criticisms of the plan.

Most states in the USA organise their health care services as a mix of private insurance schemes and the public funding of services for those people unable to purchase insurance. Having regard to the growing demands on state expenditure for health care, the Oregon legislature decided to withdraw public funding for organ transplants, basing this decision on the high cost, the relatively few patients involved and the limited success in terms of health gain as a result of transplantation. When a 7-year-old boy died because his parents could not afford to pay for the full cost of the operation, the media publicity that followed forced the federal government to order the restoration of transplants across the USA for everyone aged under 21 years.

The Oregon Senate was still resolved to establish some form of *explicit rationing*. At the same time, it wished to extend the Medicaid scheme for poor families by including as eligible for public funding everyone whose income fell below the official federal (central) poverty line. Within this scheme, the legislators decided to draw up a list of treatments linked to diseases that would be funded from the public purse and a list of those which would not attract public funding. In order to devise such a list, a collaborative exercise was embarked upon in which professional judgements and public preferences were to be combined in order to identify all those conditions and treatments which were considered to be of relatively high priority. The basis of the eventual 'formula' was cost-utility analysis using quality adjusted life-years (QALYs) as a measure of outcome.

A telephone survey was carried out and public meetings were held in order to consult the public about what values they attached to certain health states. Eventually – after a number of revisions – a final list was drawn up, and where there were areas of uncertainty over the 'correct' values assigned to certain functional impairments by the public, the members of the Oregon Health Services Commission made the final decision. The list consisted of 709 conditions, and treatments, and the State of Oregon decided to fund the first 587 items on the list.

Criticisms of the Oregon plan

1. The public meetings were attended predominantly by middle-class citizens, many of whom actually worked in the health care services. This sample was thus regarded by many as unrepresentative.
2. The complexity of many physical and mental conditions was not reflected in the list of items. Conditions appear as if they are exclusive of other illnesses; that is, there is no recognition of co-morbidity.
3. Many estimates of health care outcome were made entirely by clinicians even though the benefits that followed from certain treatments were neither entirely understood nor agreed, in terms of either duration or quality of life criteria.
4. The calculation of the costs involved in treatment was based on range of costs rather than particular costs *per treatment*.

Priority-setting and the public: an initiative in England

One key issue in health care planning, largely as a consequence of the publicity that the Oregon approach attracted, is the extent to which members of the public on a collective level should be invited and encouraged to play a part in deciding where resources should be directed. This debate is not, however, a completely new phenomenon. Many years ago, the WHO declared as a global policy that ordinary citizens should be involved in the process of planning for the provision of health services (WHO 1946).

One illuminative case study that has implemented this policy has been reported with regard to the establishment of local panels in the English county of Somerset, where eight health panels have been set up, each consisting of 12 people representing as far as possible a cross-section of the population, with men and women of all ages and backgrounds (Bowie *et al.* 1995). The topics for each meeting are usually proposed by the health authority. These are 'live' issues of genuine concern to the authority, and sufficient background information is given to each panel member well before each meeting, for which they are paid a small attendance fee. The meetings are facilitated by an expert in group dynamics. Some of the questions for discussion are listed below:

1. Should coronary bypass operations be denied to all smokers?
2. Should *second* bypass operations be denied to smokers who have refused to give up smoking?
3. Should the health authority pay for treatment for all sports injuries?
4. Should people with terminal cancer and less than 6 months to live be given intensive treatment or simply kept free from pain and suffering?
5. Should a fee be charged for the hospital car service for those who are medically fit to travel?
6. Should the waiting times for general surgery be 10 months, 8 months or 6 months?
7. How should the following be prioritised: paediatric nurse specialists; cancer nurses; additional cataract operations; clinical genetics; additional chiropody; and an improved drug service?
8. Should more night medical centres be set up to save on GPs' visiting time and costs?

Criticisms could be made of certain aspects of this exercise in public participation. Is it acceptable, for example, that the health authority should almost always 'set the agenda' for discussion. Is it logical to try to make judgements about prioritising completely different types of health care intervention? Does listing items in order of priority clearly indicate the value attached to each of those items by the respondents?

According to Bowie *et al.*, doctors remain sceptical with respect to the relevance of panel decision-making on resource allocation. Nevertheless, the panels' collective views have been taken seriously by the health authority, and their adjudications have influenced planning decisions. Proponents of greater public participation would argue that ordinary members of the public have – as tax-payers – a right to be consulted about where their money is being spent. In addition, difficult decisions about prioritising are more likely to be accepted if representatives of the public have contributed to those decisions. Opponents, on the other hand, could say that medical staff, perhaps in conjunction with senior managers, should not relinquish their responsibility to reach decisions that are central to planning by off-loading those decisions on to people who are unlikely to possess sufficient knowledge and expertise to come to valid judgements.

Summary

There are clearly methodological and ethical problems associated with any rationing or prioritising process. The traditional process in many countries has been one of implicit prioritising, that is, the allocation of priorities being made by doctors in deciding who will receive swift treatment and who will go on a waiting list. A decision actually to refuse treatment is one that most doctors would find ethically unacceptable. Yet decisions of this nature – concerning which treatments for which conditions will be funded, partly funded or not funded at all, at the public's expense – are becoming commonplace in many health care systems.

The Oregon plan is only one approach to the recurring problem of planning health care services in a way that will manage a balance between equity and value for money. There are countries that provide 'free' health care for everyone at the point of need, although such a system usually co-exists with private health care paid for by insurance cover and/or payment in part at the point of service. Planning in order to match resources to demand or to shape demand to the resources available is not a function that can be detached from issues relating to funding in other areas: on a macro level, for example, the ratio of total budgets on health, defence, education, social welfare, and so on; on a micro level, the ratio of expenditure on health care services to the money dedicated to research, staffing, training and administration.

Dramatic advances over the past 20 years or so in the development of highly expensive surgical treatments and pharmaceutical drugs have created a demand for health care services that is of great concern to governments in developed countries. Health care planning has become a function of governments and a variety of health care organisations that is challenging and complicated. Balancing moral questions of human rights, of individual and collective interests and economic considerations, is a task that involves complex deliberations.

Items for discussion

> 1. What do you consider to be the advantages of and potential problems in trying to involve the public in decisions relating to health care planning?
> 2. What are the ethical and practical considerations to be borne in mind in trying to prevent health problems by encouraging people to adopt healthier lifestyles?

Chapter 7 Different approaches to health care planning

It is hard to imagine that anyone would oppose the *principles* underlying health care planning. Planning, being essentially the structured implementation of policy, would seem to be essential in order primarily to:

- Maximise the possibility that priorities can be balanced and put into effect within available resources
- Control costs
- Provide a sound basis for measuring and monitoring performance against specific targets within a clear timeframe.

In this chapter, different approaches to health care planning and critiques of these approaches will be presented. The word 'critique' is, however, neutral: it is a critical analysis that may be positive, negative or include elements of both. Adverse comments about health care planning are not likely to be focused on the purpose or intention but on other considerations, for example:

- The *means or methods* for achieving the aims of planning
- The *value context* in which techniques of planning are based
- The *model of health* that provides the framework for planning activities
- The extent to which health care planning is *achieving its objectives*.

Another issue that might lead to negative comments about systems of health care planning is whether targets set within a specified time limit are too easy or too difficult to achieve. We shall deal with all these matters in the course of this chapter.

Techniques used in health care planning

Coast *et al.* (1996) deal comprehensively with a variety of technical approaches to the first objective of planning, which has to do with developing some 'equation' between needs, demand and resources. We shall give only brief references here. Each technique has its merits and defects, each constitutes a means or method of planning, and each can be combined with an other or others in the process of planning for health care services.

Programme budgeting and marginal analysis

Health authorities and health care organisations must first decide which programmes are relevant to their strategy in terms of disease groups or specialties. These 10–20 programmes must be capable of being costed with a reasonable degree of accuracy. Each programme is then inspected to see whether any reallocations of resources within the programme could bring about an increase in benefits; that is marginal (small-scale) changes are analysed using primarily cost–benefit analysis. This process can then be applied not only within particular programmes, but also across all the programmes.

Equity and needs assessment

'Equity' refers to equal access to health care for those in equal need. The basis of equal access for equal need could involve meeting all the greatest needs and none of the lesser ones, or the setting up of some provision for all needs but less provision for lesser needs. There are two types of 'equity' in economists' models:

1. *Vertical equity*: treating differently those with different needs
2. *Horizontal equity*: treating equally those people with the same or very similar needs.

The assessment of needs within a health context could, in itself, be the subject matter of an extended discussion. Diagnosis is not an exact science, and clinical judgements on the actual medical condition and the most efficacious intervention may vary. Apart from this potential problem, how governments and health authorities create or encourage 'equal access' is not straightforward because of the co-existence in many countries of public and private avenues to services.

Age-based rationing

The justification for this approach to resource planning is that each individual would, in theory, have a greater benefit over their lifetime if the resources currently used to extend life were instead used earlier in life. Age is used as a criterion for choosing who should receive care.

Supporters of this approach argue that making this criterion explicit would be more open and honest than using age as a criterion in 'implicit rationing'. Coast *et al.* (1996), citing a number of references, draw attention to the relatively low rates of renal dialysis treatment and coronary care for patients above a certain age.

The value context

The fact that health care planning takes place to any degree in various countries indicates an involvement by the government in the provision of health care services. This means that access to health care is not left exclusively to the market. For whatever reason or reasons, the planning of the resourcing and delivery of health care services by governments and their agencies reflects an obligation on the part of governments to intervene.

Exactly *what* form such intervention takes will depend on the prevailing values on which the government or agency considers itself legitimised to act. A *collective* approach will attempt to spread resources evenly in order to achieve the greatest benefit for the greatest number. A *discriminatory* strategy could direct more resources per head into a region or area that is experiencing higher than average levels of morbidity, or could lead to decisions not to offer expensive treatment for individuals who have ignored medical advice or whose lifestyle has directly led to a condition requiring costly, invasive surgery.

Here again, the issue of explicit versus implicit rationing is relevant. On ethical grounds, in accordance with the Hippocratic oath for example, medical practitioners should not refuse treatment on any discriminatory grounds. In practice, decisions about which patients should have prior access to care services are continuously being made. The triage system – or a variation of it – is applied in accident and emergency departments. The original locus for using this approach was the battlefield, where decisions about medical treatment were based on the relative likelihood of survival. 'Triage' is a term derived from the French word meaning 'to separate or to pick out; to sift'. Resources are, in this scenario, allocated to those cases that are likely to show the most beneficial effect rather than to where the need is most urgent or severe.

Decisions of this nature have to be made in those situations where a number of sick people are awaiting the opportunity for an organ transplant. Who should receive the liver or heart? In certain cultures, of course, this question would be answered by a clear response, namely that no transplants should be permitted because of prevailing beliefs about the nature of the human body and of life itself.

Models of 'health' and health care

In many parts of the world, public health medicine, with its emphasis on tackling health problems through the prevention and early detection of illness at the community level, has given way to the mainstream biomedical approach, which focuses more narrowly on the manifestation, diagnosis and treatment of disease in individuals (Baggott 1998). There are, however, some signs that a revival of the public health approach is gaining ground in developed countries. In less-developed parts of the globe, the emphasis is still likely to be on preventive and health promotion measures.

The dominant perspective in Western culture of regarding the body and mind as distinct entities has also contributed to the development of health care interventions that are, in essence, fragmented. We acknowledge in Western societies the probable psychosomatic influence on the aetiology and 'career' of certain pathological conditions, but the vast array of specialties that has been created in conventional medicine and the predominantly hospital-based context of treatment clearly articulates not only an information base, but also an interpretation of the body as a quasi-mechanical entity amenable, hopefully, to remedial interventions.

In the West, the growing profile of alternative or complementary medicine reflects an unease with this dominant biomedical model of illness. In other quarters, too, such as in Eastern societies, the traditional modes of dealing with health and illness may co-exist alongside the biomedical model (Freund and McGuire 1991).

Critical perspectives √

From the points of view of different interest groups in society, health care planning reveals a commitment to a particular ideology that they might not share. We have referred at the outset to the distinction between health planning and health care planning. The former concept acknowledges the complex factors that are responsible for an individual's, a community's or a nation's health status. These can be broadly described as environmental factors such as sanitation, water supplies and air-borne pollution that can have a direct bearing on health, as well as other social experiences, for example poor standards of housing, homelessness and long-term unemployment, which appear to be correlated with relatively high morbidity rates (Baggott 1998).

In July 1998 in the UK, the Chancellor of the Exchequer announced that an additional £2 billion was to be allocated to the NHS over a period of 3 years, money earmarked for the building of new hospitals. A main consideration influencing this decision was the government's election manifesto promise to reduce hospital waiting lists for treatment. Six months after this budgetary announcement, at February 1999 (the time of writing this chapter), the number on waiting lists had risen by nearly 12 per cent, to well over a million would-be patients.

Such a policy can be legitimately interpreted as overemphasising the role of secondary and tertiary care at the expense of primary care. Furthermore, the funding for additional hospitals means that resources are likely to be diverted from improving those environmental and social factors that are seen by many – the UK government included – as contributing to the poorer health of people who are on a relatively low level of income.

At the root of adverse criticism about health and health care planning is a sense of discrimination. The negative connotation signifies that planning of services accepts the inevitability, if not the desirability, of inequity – that some sections of society are likely to lose out in the strategic distribution of resources. We shall examine the critiques articulated from three perspectives, drawing on the work of Baggott (1998).

The socialist perspective

Perhaps the most influential ideological critique of social discrimination has been the Marxist thesis. In their analysis of health care systems, proponents of this world view would identify inequalities in the provision of health care as a feature of capitalism, inequalities being greater in countries where private enterprise plays a major role in the provision of services. Where there is greatest need for resources, in areas of relatively high material deprivation, one might expect governments to respond by discriminating *positively*, encouraging more doctors to work in such areas and removing some of the barriers to improved health such as substandard housing and unemployment. Tudor-Hart (1971), a very experienced GP who established a practice in a very deprived area of South Wales, has characterised the actual situation as the *inverse law* of resource allocation: those who need most get least. From the Marxist viewpoint, the fault lies with the prevailing political ideology and the social system that flows from it:

Marxists believe that the health care system is a microcosm of the capitalist society in which it operates. They see a clear class bias in the production of health care. For them, the upper classes and upper-middle classes are in a position to decide on key questions of resource allocation and the organisation of care. State health care systems operating within capitalist societies are not regarded as special cases. (Baggott 1998, p. 72)

Countries committed to the principles enunciated by WHO (1978) will be planning their service provision so that every citizen has access to at least basic health care services irrespective of his or her income. The Marxist critique, Baggott argues, is too fundamentalist and ignores the reality that capitalist societies, with all the shortcomings of social inequalities, make genuine efforts to subsidise the health care of poorer people. The Marxist response would be that any effort to improve the health of the workers is a means towards the end of enhanced capitalistic profit-making.

The feminist critique

Objections to the role assigned to women in health care systems have been expressed under three broad categories:

1. Employment within health care settings
2. Assumptions about their role as carers
3. Experience as patients.

We have come some way in most societies from the historical prejudices about women as medical practitioners that found an exponent in one American physician (quoted in Wertz and Wertz 1979):

the periodical infirmity of their sex... in every case... unfits them for any responsible effort of mind... [and that during their menstrual] condition, neither life nor limb submitted to them would be as safe as at other times. (p. 57)

Yet the prestigious and politically influential medical profession is still universally male dominated, and nurses remain largely disempowered as the female 'handmaidens' of doctors.

Planning health services relies to a large extent on a dependence on traditional social and cultural expectations of women's role as family carers. This assumption can account, at least in part, for the relatively low priority accorded to primary health care in many countries. Deakin (1987) noted that feminist critiques of community care policy reflected the way in which care in the community contributed to the oppression of women by reinforcing gendered assumptions about caring roles and added to the emotional and material burdens of many women who had to combine both paid work and unpaid informal caring. The comparative costing of community care as opposed to institutional care has often omitted to calculate the *opportunity costs* involved when female carers give up work in order to look after heavily dependent family members.

In 1979, Doyal and Gough argued that doctors adopt a view of female health problems that is often linked with prevailing ideas about their reproductive role. If doctors assume that motherhood and the maternal instinct are the major driving force in women's lives, one possible consequence is to interpret a variety of female health problems as having their origins in a denial of this instinct. Miles (1988) gathered evidence that doctors are more likely to diagnose women as being neurotically and emotionally imbalanced than men who exhibit similar presenting problems.

Roberts (1992) produced evidence to indicate that the medical profession has failed to take account of the particular needs of women when planning and delivering services. A notable example is childbirth, in which it is claimed that the medical dominance of procedures has led to the subjugation of women in treating childbirth as a form of illness rather than a natural condition.

The disability movement

The WHO (1980) has produced an important checklist that identifies the attributes of impairment, disability and handicap, which are defined by the *International Classification of Impairments, Disabilities and Handicaps* (ICIDH).

Impairments are regarded as 'any loss or abnormality of psychological, physiological or anatomical structure or function'. These comprise intellectual, language, aural, ocular, visceral, skeletal, disfiguring, other psychological and generalised, and sensory impairments. Disability and handicap are treated by the ICIDH as the functional and social consequences of impairment.

A *disability* refers to 'failures of accomplishment'; a *handicap* is distinguished as being 'the disadvantages experienced by an individual as a result of impairments and disabilities'. According to these conceptual distinctions, neither disability nor handicap necessarily follows as a result of an impairment. For example, a person who has to wear spectacles may not suffer any problem carrying out tasks such as personal care, communicating with other people and performing tasks calling for a degree of dexterity, and would also be unlikely to experience any handicap other than perhaps being ineligible to become an airline pilot. Conversely, left-handed people – although not impaired – might feel a sense of disability in what is predominantly a right-handed world.

Advocates of disabled persons' rights resent the fact that society is organised to the detriment and disadvantage of people with what might broadly be termed 'physical disabilities'. Far from ensuring, through policies founded on the principle of positive discrimination, that those with various impairments are enabled to function socially and occupationally on a par with non-impaired people, most societies are culpable of what Townsend (1962) has defined as *structured dependency*. A lack of access to buildings, to public transport and to jobs is an example of the way in which policies often disadvantage impaired and disabled individuals.

In order to move towards social and occupational parity with non-disabled persons, those with disabilities resulting from impairments would wish to see health and health care planners adopt a wider vision than one based on the medical objectives of *care* and *cure*. Pressure groups involving disabled people are active in many countries and have a common aim: to influence attitudes towards planning that emphasises a medical rather than a social model of the concepts of 'disability' and 'handicap'. In 1990, Disabled Peoples International was formed. This is accepted by the United Nations as the only legitimate representative organisation of disabled people (Oliver 1997).

Until recently, even with the efforts of voluntary groups, social attitudes towards impaired people have subscribed to a form of 'social Darwinism' – an acceptance that impairment and its resulting disabilities and handicaps are part and parcel of the human condition just as some creatures will survive or thrive by being more capable of adapting to external circumstances. In terms of the WHO definition of 'health' as a state of complete physical, mental and social well-being, most societies seem to be doing very little to create structural and attitudinal change that will drastically reduce the need for disabled people to adopt a marginalised social role.

All three critiques of health care policy and planning raise issues about the way in which poor, female and impaired individuals are forced into a position of disadvantage because of prevailing capitalist, male-dominated cultures.

Other critiques of health care planning

According to Green (1995):

one of the problems that planning has faced over the last two decades is its own poor record in achieving change. (p. 23)

A purely technocratic approach to health care planning, in which problems are identified and technical means of solving or relieving them are implemented, ignores the *political* nature of planning. Green points to a number of possible reasons why there has been a gap between setting objectives and actually achieving them:

Decentralisation

This has often occurred without careful consideration of the relative roles and functions of the centre and the periphery in the planning process. The centre's role is to provide broad strategic guidelines, to make allocative decisions regarding resources, to co-ordinate local plans and to provide specialist planning advice. The periphery's (that is agency's) role is to develop and implement local plans. 'However, the longer such roles are left unclear, the harder it is for planning to be re-established' (Green 1995, p. 25).

The rise of non-government organisations

Non-government organizations (NGOs) constitute a relatively fragmented sector. However, as donors shift their attention to this sector and put resources into it, the growth in the size of the sector suggests the need for more, rather than fewer, co-ordination and regulatory mechanisms.

Short-termism

On the one hand, there is an understandable impatience to see a real improvement in health status; on the other, there are pressures relating to the needs of politicians and professionals in donor agencies to demonstrate results.

Setting targets

Targets are specific, usually quantitative goals to be achieved within a particular period. Targets spelt out by the WHO have influenced similar exercises in many parts of the world: governments have produced plans in which such aims as the reduction of certain morbidity and mortality rates linked to key diseases have been earmarked for action. Such targets need to be realistic and meaningful; in addition, there have to be mechanisms in place to monitor the means by which the targets will be reached and to ensure that, if targets *are* reached, there is evidence to prove that such changes can be unequivocally related to the expressed means. For example, can it be proved that a health promotion campaign designed to reduce the incidence of breast cancer by a given percentage has been directly responsible for any such decrease in cases?

It is also crucial to discover why targets have not been reached. Were the targets themselves unrealistic, were external circumstances responsible, or did funding suddenly decrease? Some of this analysis is similar in its application to questions surrounding policy implementation (see Chapter 4). For targets to be meaningful, they have to herald some significant and measurable achievement if they are met. There is hardly any purpose in setting targets that might be attained merely with the passage of time. For example, some physical problems might improve through 'watchful waiting' and non-intervention.

Planning for distant scenarios

In Chapter 6 reference was made to 'future studies'. These are exercises in long-term forecasts of health care demands based on what might be termed extensive Delphi panel consultation. The Welsh Health Planning Forum, for example, was very active during the 1980s and 90s, drawing upon the informed opinions of a range of experts in the field of health in order to depict a society's health care needs nearly 20 years into the future. This form of 'crystal ball' planning has to have a foundation of informed expert opinion, current data on epidemiological and demographic trends and a precondition of relative political and economic stability. A key document (Welsh Health Planning Forum, 1992) based its predictions – as all studies of this longitudinal perspective have to do – on sound, accurate information. The premises on which the planning was based were these:

● People will be less willing to accept ill-health and will become more demanding consumers of health services.

- People will feel greater empowerment. They will be given more information as patients and will be encouraged to participate in the planning of their own care.
- Health needs will change with the population structure and patterns of disease.
- The role of hospitals will change as the length of inpatient stay falls and more care is provided at home.
- Primary care will face new challenges with shifts in the location of services and in consumer expectations.
- There will be a growing need for partnership between health and social services, and between statutory and voluntary agencies.

Acknowledging that 'we cannot predict the future but we can envisage how it might be' (p. 5), the report sets out specific benchmarks derived from current data. This is a selection:

- All mental illness and mental handicap hospitals should be closed.
- Everyone over 85 years old should have a key worker.
- 15 per cent of births will take place outside hospital.
- 80 per cent of surgical interventions should be bloodless by 2002.
- 60 per cent of surgery should be day case by 2002.

The report goes on to deal with 'levers of change' such as financial arrangements, existing structures, professional skills and attitudes, public attitudes, expectations and information.

The use of the word 'should' in this context is ambiguous. Does it mean 'is likely to happen', or is it indicating what *ought* to happen? A further section of the report makes it clear that health care planning is inescapably informed not only by quantitative data, but also by sets of values. Under the heading 'A Philosophy for the Future', the following principles are articulated:

Services should–

- offer real choices to users
- be as close to home as possible
- employ staff who are responsive to users
- offer continuity of care and seamless care
- use the correct level of expertise at every stage. (p. 3)

Planning services can never be an exact exercise. As this report asserts, there is always the possibility of unforeseen health problems occurring, for example another Chernobyl-type incident or the resurgence of 'old' problems such as tuberculosis. It is also hazardous to rule out the possibility of an economic crisis on a scale experienced during the late 1990s in the Far East, which can undermine the long-term plans of governments. Future studies rely on a combination of several potentially conflicting components in order to make authoritative statements:

1. Statistical data, for example population and disease patterns
2. Calculations relating to future demand
3. Assumptions about shared values
4. Expert opinions on key developments such as the application of technology and its impact on treatments and costs
5. Political awareness concerning the likelihood of key policies being maintained or changed in the event of a change of government.

Summary

Although the key yardstick by which to judge the value of planning is perhaps the extent to which the health of the population, or targeted sections of the population, has improved as a result, health care planning can also be justified by reference to the way in which it contributes to the whole system of decision-making, particularly with regard to resource allocation.

Is 'planning' at the opposite extreme to 'muddling through', as Lindblom depicted the process and practice of decision-making? It would certainly seem to be so whenever 3-, 5- or even 10-year plans are produced. Even though the demands of political reality will tend towards foreshortening the time-horizon for the 'structured implementation of policy', there is no doubt that the act of planning implies a carefully considered, albeit flexible, attempt at reducing uncertainty in the allocation of resources.

Although it is natural to think of planning as a systematic method of putting policy into operation, the very act of devising future scenarios for longer-term health and health care planning may be helpful in shaping policies. Planning, in this context, may *precede* policy. The various critiques presented above challenge any assumptions that planning is a process that is instrumentally neutral in the sense that it is value-free. From the political perspective of the left, from the feminist point of view and from that of disability movements, health care planning reveals an ideological underpinning that reflects dominant political ideologies. Resource allocation decisions that have to be made within a framework of broad policy, such as the move towards care and treatment outside hospital, are influenced by the relative importance attached by policy-makers to the claims of different patient groups and to different forms of care and treatment. Another example of health and health care planning being driven by dominant interests is the prioritising of certain programmes above others by donors when they grant funding to developing countries.

There is evidence for suggesting that governments can be highly selective in apportioning resources not only on the basis of proven health needs, but also in response to political demands. They may also be selective in the data that they choose in order to make planning decisions. The foundation on which planning has to be built is a sound information base that includes not only 'hard' data but also the softer, more qualitative indicators of public opinion and personal perceptions in such areas as health care outcomes. In the next two chapters, we deal with the question of information for planning.

Items for discussion

1. In what ways can *discrimination* be both a positive and negative influence on the planning of health care services?
2. Consider the question of *values* as a major issue in health care planning.

Chapter 8 Information needs for health care planning – I

It is important to distinguish between *information* and *data*. 'Data' refers to what might be termed 'raw evidence' collected by a variety of means. A distinction is made between *hard data* and *soft data*. The former is quantitative in nature and is usually labelled as statistics; soft data are the kinds of data, for example opinions, beliefs and attitudes, that are not in themselves quantifiable numerically even though the frequency and intensity with which they are expressed can often be presented in a quantitative manner. For example, we could read that 35 per cent or 75 per cent of people interviewed believed that the government was doing a good job.

For data to become information, a number of stages have to be worked through. The data must be *categorised*, that is, put into some form of classification system. The data also have to be *analysed* – sorted into some 'order' or 'pattern'. This imposition of order upon data is crucial. It enables the next stage – the *interpretation* of the data – to be carried out. By this process, we move from the question, What data do we have?, through to the next stages, which seek answers to the question, What data can be grouped together as similar?, and on to the final question, What does it all mean? 'Information' is data to which there are attached some meaning and significance for those who interpret it.

The politics of data

Some data are undeniably accurate and comprehensive. The number of days in a week, the number of degrees in a circle – these are 'statistics' that are given and accepted. Problems arise when data are subjected to analysis and interpretation using another factor or *variable* as a reference point. For example, there may be no dispute over a hospital's records that show a 10 per cent decrease in the length of stay in a particular ward over a period of 6 months, but what these data *mean* is a more complex issue. To the administrator, this might mean that a gain in throughput efficiency has been achieved; to a senior nurse, the figures might indicate a poorer quality of patient care.

The point being made here is, perhaps, obvious: transforming data into information involves the application of different perspectives, and these different perspectives will be shaped by different 'criteria', which will, in turn, be influenced by different 'values'. It is common knowledge that people in powerful positions may release data only selectively to the public at large in order to further their own political interests; workers within an organisation may be kept 'in the dark' by management. Data can be suppressed or manipulated by civil servants and public administrators so that politicians who have the legislative authority come to conclusions that suit the aspirations of these senior personnel.

What follows from this description of 'data' and 'information' is that reality is a *relative* concept when we are discussing the merits and de-merits of health care services. Facts and figures may be flawed because of the suspect or inadequate methods used in order to assemble the data; or they may be deceptive because they are being presented selectively and in a biased manner; or, as we have noted above, the data may be accepted by everyone as 'facts', but there may be a good deal of variation in the way in which these 'facts' are interpreted.

Figure 8.1 demonstrates this point. Mortality statistics can be assumed to be accurate since the recording of deaths is systematic and comprehensive.

The quantitative data in Figure 8.1 give us some information about the relative death rate of a proportion of the general population (ethnic group Z) compared with the total population. For health care policy-makers and planners, however, these basic data are not enough because they do not *explain* why there is a difference between certain sections of the population. Questions of equity arise. In order to enhance social justice by narrowing the gap between the health states of various social 'strata', more data are required that could indicate why such differences are found.

SMR = Actual deaths over expected deaths x 100

For example, in a given population, the prevalence of deaths can be expressed according to ethnic group, social class, sex or some other classification.

Ethnic group Z:

No. in population (A)	Death rate per 1000 (total population) (B)	Expected deaths (A x B)
40 000	30	1200

Actual deaths in ethnic group Z = 1500

$$\text{SMR} = \frac{1500}{1200} \times 100 = 125$$

Since the death rate is higher than 100, this indicates that ethnic group Z is relatively unhealthy compared with the general population.

Figure 8.1   Standardised mortality ratio (SMR)

Without any additional data at this stage, we could draw several hypothetical inferences in order to 'explain' why people in ethnic group Z enjoy comparatively poor health compared with the population as a whole. For example, we could argue that they:

● Are genetically disposed towards worse health
● Are less health conscious and lead unhealthier lifestyles
● Are relatively poor and therefore suffer from more stress-related illness
● Are less likely to consult a doctor in order to prevent illness and remedy health problems at an early stage
● Are unable to 'jump queues' and pay privately for consultation and treatment.

None of these hypotheses can be confirmed or refuted without additional data, and it is the particular concern of epidemiologists and social scientists to search for further evidence in order to establish a relationship between two or more variables. Ideally, scientists seek to establish a cause-and-effect relationship between variables, for example between a pathological condition and the factor that directly causes that condition. In technical terms, this quest concerns *aetiology*, the study of the causes of disease. However, before this stage has been reached, the attempt to isolate one factor linked to a specific disease – or to a lack of that disease – may result in one or more factors being identified as showing a certain strength of correlation with the disease or its absence.

Data, information and decision-making

It is easy to see why decision-makers within the health and health care fields are reluctant to base any decisions on partial data that go no further than suggesting possible correlations between a variety of factors or even between one factor and a disease. Proof rather than probability should be the test of accurate information on which resource allocation can be based. This statement, however, is something of a counsel of perfection, first, because absolute proof cannot always be obtained, and second, because key decision-makers might choose to disregard such proof even if it were available.

These issues are especially relevant where ecological factors are cited as having an influence on morbidity or mortality rates. Isolating one bacterium in a research laboratory as the cause of disease 'X' might be open to less political controversy than data suggesting a link between a relatively high prevalence of asthma among certain individuals and their proximity to busy highways or industrial plants. The apparent delay in acknowledging the link between 'mad cow disease' and certain foodstuffs given to the affected animals, and the consequent debate in the UK about the possible link between the human consumption of contaminated beef and Creutzfeldt–Jacob disease underline the complexity of decision-making.

The matrix of interrelated components influencing policy-making described in Chapter 1 applies throughout the process of policy and planning, and the question of what evidence is *politically acceptable* highlights the deficiencies of both the rational and incremental models of decision-making. The term 'politically acceptable' is used here to mean acceptable to the dominant political group, and this criterion of acceptability might, in turn, be defined according to the perceived political repercussions of a decision that does or does not find favour with other interest groups such as the business sector, trade unions and the electorate.

Neither the comprehensive rationality nor bounded rationality models of Simon (1957), nor the disjointed incrementalism model articulated by Lindblom (1959), fully acknowledges the issue of competing rationalities inherent in the processes of policy and planning decisions. For example, the data might clearly be stating that, in any one country, the disparity in health states is strongly correlated with level of income and, consequently, with lifestyle and living conditions forced upon the less fortunate members of society. An acceptance of these facts would not necessarily lead to government action in order to redress the imbalance between rich and poor. Ideological commitment to self-help rather than state intervention; a fiscal policy that seeks to reduce public expenditure; an assessment of the political consequences within the country and externally if a particular course of action is pursued – all of these considerations could provide an entirely logical argument for doing nothing. The only model that could serve as being universally applicable to all macro decision-making is one that stresses political survival as the central core.

The main argument for developing sophisticated information systems and accurate databases is to enhance the quality of decision-making. This might appear to contradict the thesis developed in the previous section – that political concerns are at the heart of decision-making. In this context, the contribution of data and information to the policy-making process has been subjected to scrutiny, and, in doing so, we have noted that however compelling the evidence might be for more resources, for example to be allocated in a positively discriminating way in order to offset social injustices, decision makers have the power to make logical choices that do not necessarily accord with the preferred options of various interest groups. Data and information generated in order to implement stated policy objectives are used in order to help to answer strictly operational questions. To this end, planning is a systematic approach to minimising future uncertainties.

Neuberger (1994) has listed various types of data needed for health care planning:

- Epidemiological data, including variance in the incidence of disease locally, regionally nationally and internationally
- Comparative health care outcomes data

- Risk versus benefit analysis, for example on procedures and drugs
- Clinical profiles of care
- The results of research, including randomised control trials
- Social, economic and environmental determinants of health.

We shall add to this list later on. Here, Neuberger is referring to planning more at a macro/strategic level than at a functional/operational level, although some of the types of data, such as the last example, could equally be relevant to more localised planning.

Health indicators

The WHO have developed a number of 'health indicators' in order to help countries to monitor their progress towards the targets of *Health for All by the Year 2000* (WHO 1985).

1. *Health status*
   - Morbidity and mortality rates

2. *Health care provision*
   - Availability, for example the ratio of doctors and health centres per total population
   - Accessibility – physical (location) and economic (affordability)
   - Utilisation – actual coverage and usage, for example the proportion of pregnant women who receive antenatal care or the percentage of children being immunised

3. *Health policy*
   - Resource allocation – the proportion of the gross national product spent on health services, primary health care and public health. Equity of distribution of resources geographically or by patient group.

Social indicators

'Social indicators' are a means of counterbalancing exclusively economic measures as being indicative of social well-being. The logical basis for gathering data under this heading is that factors such as long-term unemployment, low income, substandard housing and a poor physical environment are correlated with relatively high levels of morbidity and mortality. All these phenomena can be summarised by the term 'social deprivation', which is a form of social pathology. Because of the complexity of isolating these different factors in a quasi-experimental research design, it is virtually impossible to establish a cause-and-effect link between symptoms of social deprivation and illnesses. Nevertheless, there is substantial evidence, in terms of 'hard data' supported by the 'soft data' derived from interviews with people living in these areas, that 'relative deprivation' (frequently used as a euphemism for 'poverty') leads to a deterioration in health.

Epidemiological data

The study of the distribution of disease and disability and of the factors that influence that distribution may be described as a form of medical ecology. Epidemiologists are concerned with *states*, that is identifying sets of attributes, for example the number with certain disabilities and diseases, and with *events* such as accidents, changes in health state, illness episodes and trends over time.

The practice of epidemiology will focus on the geographical distribution of illnesses, seasonal cycles, contact patterns, proximity patterns regarding sources of hazard, behavioural disorders such as heroin addiction, and iatrogenic disease, for example the side-effects of drugs and the effects of medical error. Data collection can essentially be divided into two categories:

1. *Prevalence*: the general distribution of disease at any given time
2. *Incidence*: the number of new cases within a particular period.

Epidemiological data contribute to health care planning because they help to expose correlations between phenomena in the external environment and the impairment of health, and because they enable predictions to be made about trends and incidences of diseases in a given locality. Decisions on where to direct resources and what types of intervention might be necessary can then be made with greater clarity.

101

Hospital-based data

The range and types of data collected by hospital managers/administrators are wide and will probably include most or all of the following:

- The use of inpatient facilities, for example hospital admissions, bed-days, bed occupancy and the duration of stay and discharges
- Surgical operations, including day surgery and anaesthetic procedures
- Outpatient attendances at specialist clinics, accident and emergency departments and dental clinics
- Radiological and laboratory investigations and the extent of the use of services provided by physiotherapists and occupational therapists
- The use of pharmaceutical products
- Community nursing services
- Health screening and immunisation
- Patient disease statistics including mortality data
- Detailed patient profiles
- Hospital personnel records and workload indicators.

In some situations, such as a quasi-market or internal market culture within a health care system (for example the UK), hospitals will also be using *performance indicators* (see below) to monitor what might broadly be termed 'efficiency of performance', as well as *outcome measures*, for example the costs and 'success rates' of various treatments. The whole area of health care outcomes is of considerable and increasing importance to health service providers. We shall refer to this issue in Chapter 9.

The application of data

The data derived from the various approaches set out in previous sections contribute in a number of ways to health care planning:

- *Patient sickness records* provide information necessary for the analysis of prevailing morbidity patterns and trends of diseases in the community, and help to supplement data gath-

ered from mortality records, national census data, GP notifi-
cations of communicable, notifiable diseases, and general
demographic and epidemiological data.

● *Health services utilisation statistics* contribute to the monitoring
and appraisal of the performance of various health services
and the extent of usage by patients.

● *Past morbidity and health service utilisation patterns* provide
useful inputs in making projections of probable future needs
and demands on the health service, and in mapping out
appropriate strategies to meet the anticipated changes.

● *Patient and service data* will assist in devising plans relating to
the planning of new departments, the projection of future
workforce needs, bed provision and health care costing.

Assessing need

Two key activities that depend on full and accurate information
for health care planning are the 'allocation of resources' and the
'measurement of performance'. In the next chapter, we shall
look in more detail at a range of approaches to measuring
performance in health care, although this area of concern will
be introduced later in this chapter in a discussion of performance indicators.

A central obligation of governments and of agencies with
delegated powers to organise the direct delivery of health care
services is to assess the health care needs of the population. Yet
the word 'need' is not easy to define in the context of health
care planning. To identify the *need* for food among a starving
population is to use the word in the sense of *necessity* – food is
essential in order to survive. In the typology of need devised by
Maslow (1970), human beings exhibit a 'hierarchy of needs'.
Maslow maintained that we seek first to satisfy our lowest level
needs (for *food, warmth, shelter* and *sleep*). It is only after these
needs have been met that we then try to satisfy needs of a
higher level. Figure 8.2 sets out this theory in the form of a
pyramid of needs.

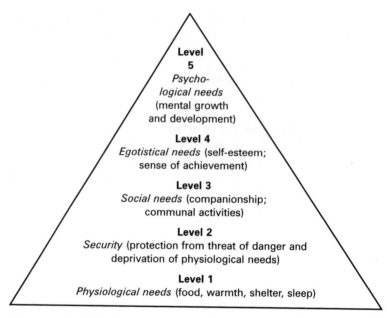

Figure 8.2   Maslow's hierarchy of needs

Maslow provides an interesting explanation of need-fulfilling desires that appear to motivate human behaviour, but the idea of 'need' is often interpreted differently by professionals who have a duty to assess what services patients should receive. The current philosophy in the UK is to establish a 'needs-led' system of integrated care services in which not only the health and social services are involved in assessment: the intended beneficiary of the services, and if appropriate his or her close family, also participates in decisions about the 'package of care' that is deemed most suitable to match their 'needs'. The language of health care and social work practitioners, however, refers to 'needs' when their real concern is in fact in identifying a *need for* specific care services in which they have a particular professional interest. Ordinary people in the street are more likely to be aware of problems that they wish to relieve, solve or prevent.

McKillip (1987) defines a need as 'a value judgement that *some group has a problem that can be solved*' (p. 10; original italics). While we could criticise this definition as apparently ignoring the importance of individual need, the author introduces the key concept of a value judgement and, in so doing, uses a personalised example:

Recognising need involves *values*. People with different values will recognise different needs. Further, the person seeing the need and the person experiencing the need may differ. An observer may judge your state of affairs inadequate, even though you yourself experience no dissatisfaction. (p. 10)

McKillip goes on to state that, in order to solve problems, a needs analysis has to be carried out, and this will rely on information about the magnitude of the problem(s) and the cost, impact and feasibility of solutions. He cites the work of Bradshaw (1972), which identifies four types of expectation that support judgements of need:

1. *Normative need*: expectation based on an expert definition of adequate levels of performance or service
2. *Felt need*: which depends on the insight that a population or individual has into a particular problem
3. *Expressed need*: expectations being reflected by the use of services, for example by waiting lists or a high bed occupancy rate
4. *Comparative need*: expectations being based on the performance of a group other than the target population, for example if one group uses services less than another or scores above or below the average, such as on dependency measure indexes.

In certain circumstances, all of the above could be criticised as offering only *prima facie* evidence of need for help of some kind. Data about waiting lists, for example, might only partly reflect a need for treatment. Further investigation might show that a percentage of those statistics relate to people whose names appear on the list as a form of 'insurance policy', for whom a service is not required immediately or even in the very near future. Averages, too, should be scrutinised carefully in order to assess the actual information that they are providing. The arithmetic mean – in which individual scores are aggregated, the sum then being divided by the total number of units – can be a particularly misleading figure on which to base decisions about resource allocation.

Even when the data are irrefutable, whether they become a trigger for action will depend on the feasibility of solving the problem. Data that demonstrate a strong correlation between poor housing and health could indicate the *need for* additional income that would enable those who live in such conditions to move into a healthier environment. A needs-led service is likely to be offered only within the constrained limits of what services are appropriate, available and accessible. Assessment of need, therefore, is predetermined by the selective use of data that filter out those elements outside the control and competence of the providing agencies. In other words, planning health care services on a one-to-one or community basis has to take place within existing policy and legislation. To an extent, it has to disregard or 'reinterpret' information that calls for action outside the sphere of health care policy itself. For example, data concerning the distribution of disease and its correlation with income level within a population or, indeed, across nations could lead to policies that set out to redistribute wealth so that income level and, as a consequence, health status might become more equitable. Health care planners have to work within existing 'global' economic policies.

In determining the role of data collection for the purposes of allocating resources, it is probably more helpful to talk about *demand* rather than need. 'Hard' data about increasingly ageing populations, greater social mobility among young people, the development and application of new medical technology and other 'facts' can assist planners to anticipate and respond to service demand. Other data, perhaps not as 'hard' as the above examples, also contribute to planning where resources should be targeted. Economic trends, the projected recruitment of health services staff and the development of new treatments to prevent and/or cure chronic and killer diseases also have to be considered. Some calculations are extremely difficult. To what extent, for example, will the supply of more doctors, nurses and advanced technology in the tertiary sector affect the demand for hospital-based health care rather than primary care? How accurate a gauge of actual health levels within any given population is the expressed demand?

According to McKillip, 'need' involves the recognition of a problem by observers. 'Need' has a more dispassionate quality than 'demand' and, because of this, is more popular with planners and academic researchers than with politicians. Demands differ from needs because the target population, rather than a service provider, usually initiates and presents a demand. Information that is provided in order to guide planning decisions about targeting resources has to be much more sophisticated than a catalogue of statistics.

Performance indicators

The word 'performance' requires close scrutiny in this context. Any indicators are, by definition, not expected to 'tell the whole story'. They provide grounds or evidence for planning but they have their limitations, as indeed do all other 'indicators of performance'. The point is, What is meant in any context by 'performance'? Performance indicators (PIs) are used in health service systems as quantifiable measures of *procedural efficiency*. The term 'efficiency' is used here in the wider sense of carrying out tasks in the minimum time and at a minimum financial cost.

PIs are stated in patients' charters, mission statements and annual planning documents and are expressed in the form of quantitative targets such as:

- 'All telephone calls from members of the public will be referred to the appropriate member(s) of staff within 3 minutes of the call being received.'
- 'All written enquiries from members of the public will receive a reply within 5 working days.'
- 'All non-complicated maternity cases will remain in hospital for no longer than 48 hours.'

Some PIs are used in order to compile sets of data not only for internal consumption by the health authority, hospital, clinic or other health care service agency, but also for inclusion in nation-wide statistics. Some particular indicators in this category could be (Harrison *et al.* 1990):

- The average number of patients per bed per year
- The average waiting time for certain operations
- The average length of stay in hospital by medical specialty
- The number of inpatient admissions per 10 000 population.

The compilation of a set of statistical data that can provide an accurate, if superficial account of what is happening nationally depends on each health authority and other relevant agencies providing data that are accurate and comprehensive. PIs founder on inadequate data and recording systems and, unless these are subjected to continuous external and internal scrutiny, there is no guarantee that the composite national statistics bear close comparison with 'reality' (Phillips *et al.* 1994).

The potential hazard of collecting data of this kind is that they might be invoked as a proxy indicator of 'quality of service'. Managerial concerns for improved efficiency are, of course, both legitimate and central in order to maximise the impact of inputs on outputs. More pernicious, perhaps, is the temptation to compare the 'performance' of hospitals or other sectors of a health service solely on the basis of quantitative data such as recovery or mortality rates for certain categories of patient. This superficial analysis ignores important variables such as the condition of the patient before the medical intervention took place, the actual *process* of care and the longer-term experiences of relative pain or discomfort after the patient has been discharged.

Summary

In this chapter, the focus has been on *quantitative data*. If we reflect upon the *system model* as a framework for policy and planning analysis, we can say that much of these data concentrate on the relationship between inputs and outputs. They also focus on procedures and throughput. Hard data of this type play a key part in producing a basis for decision-making about where finite resources should in future be targeted.

However, such data provide only a partial picture. The extent to which inputs and outputs, procedures and throughputs affect key stake-holders in health service systems remains largely unrecorded. Health care planners need other, additional data that will help to provide answers to the question, So what? What impact do all the material resources and procedures have on the intended beneficiaries, notably patients, families, communities, staff and the nation as a whole? We need, in other words, to consider means and techniques for assessing outcomes and process. These particular issues will be dealt with in Chapter 9.

Items for discussion

1. Consider the various sources of statistical data that could be relevant for health care planning at national and local community levels.
2. Comparative data show that the USA spends a much greater percentage of its gross domestic product on health care than any other nation. What hypothetical inferences can be drawn from this statistic?

Chapter 9   Information needs for health care planning – II

In several countries in recent years, there has been a disquiet with purely clinical assessments of health care interventions. We have already noted that, from a health administrator's perspective, issues such as efficiency and cost-effectiveness have come to the forefront as an essential criterion of the measurement of 'performance'. Certainly, in those health care systems where there are opportunities to 'play the market' in purchasing services, the providers of those services have entered a competitive arena where many individuals and corporate agencies such as health authorities and primary care practices are seeking value for money.

The term 'value for money' is not easy to define. Rather like the concept of 'quality', it is perhaps used without pausing to consider how its interpretation might vary from one health care stake-holder to the next. Conventionally, 'value for money' has to do with the relationship between inputs and outputs. It is a matter of comparing cost with the nature of the 'product' or 'service'. Unlike the situation in the marketplace, however, consumers of care services rarely have the opportunity to make comparisons between the services provided by different agencies. That is why satisfaction surveys may be of only limited usefulness in attempts to evaluate the performance of health care professionals and the environment in which they offer care.

Quality control

Every trained professional working in health care organisations has an interest in providing the best possible services to the recipients of those services. Standards of professional practice do not have to be imposed from above or from outside. Professional bodies set their own codes of practice, including ethical standards, and each practitioner is expected to bear a commitment to upholding those standards. In line with this traditional ethical stance and the influence of a quality assurance approach to health care provision, various systems of audit have been developed. These systems are intended to provide rapid and continuous feedback on 'performance'.

Clinical audit

Clinical audit has been described (Glynn *et al.* 1996) as:

the systematic critical analysis of the quality of clinical care, by all those who contribute to care. It includes the procedures used for diagnosis and treatment, the use of resources and the resulting outcome and quality of life for patients. (p. 141)

Audit involves setting standards for a particular aspect of care, observing and measuring current practice, assessing how far – if at all – current practice varies from those standards and why it varies, and making changes so that future practice will meet the standards set at the beginning of the exercise. These stages of the audit are often described together as the 'audit cycle'.

In practice, audits should base their analysis on a mix of quantitative and qualitative data. For example, an assessment of the use of thrombolytic therapy for people admitted to hospital with myocardial infarction should consider the time from admission that it takes for patients to receive this therapy and, if necessary, identify the cause of any delays and remedy the problem. This would mean that the *procedures* were being subjected to internal monitoring.

Medical audit

Medical audit refers to the quality control of medical care by doctors, whereas clinical audit has a wider remit and includes an audit of the care delivered by the whole clinical team. In the UK, a report published in 1987 on perioperative death (Campling *et al.* 1990) signalled the beginning of a policy introduced in the White Paper *Working for Patients* (DoH 1989) that medical audit would be a requirement for all clinicians in the health service. Attention was focused on the effectiveness and quality of inpatient surgery. Some senior surgeons and anaesthetists had been concerned about the considerable variance in perioperative mortality rates for the same conditions treated in different hospitals or by different surgeons. As a result, consultants in health authorities were asked to participate in a confidential enquiry. The importance of having accessible data across localities and hospitals is borne out by the impact that data of this kind made in the context of perioperative mortality rates.

The extent, however, to which this form of quality control contributes to more efficient and effective practice is not yet established (Buttery *et al*. 1994). In this sphere of peer review, implementing changes as a consequence of inadequate or incompetent performance is problematic. Confidentiality, professional ethics and organisational resistance to change may conspire to impede specific remedial action (Phillips *et al*. 1994).

Medical audit as a means of improving the efficiency and quality of health and welfare of patients has been criticised (Hopkins 1981, Maynard 1991). Some of these criticisms are summarised below:

- Because medical audits are reviews by members of the same profession, their findings are confidential. There is, therefore, no opportunity for lay people – whether individually or in representative groups – to bring pressure to bear on the government or health authorities with a view to improving upon identified weaknesses.
- Intended beneficiaries of the services or competencies take no part in drawing up the criteria against which performance is to be judged.
- Peer review, therefore, has no contribution to make towards clarifying which aspects of the clinician–patient relationship should receive priority attention for future strategic and operational planning.
- Even if medical audits are able to improve clinical practice, there is no guarantee that improvements will occur in areas relevant to raising levels of patient satisfaction.

Management audit

Management audit describes the process by which management systems and procedures are appraised, with a view to identifying potential improvements and evaluating the efficiency and effectiveness of current performance. It involves both formative and summative evaluation (Glynn *et al.* 1996). Audit will identify both weaknesses and strengths, and will, therefore, look for ways of achieving improvement in a constructive rather than simply a critical way.

Management audit differs from internal management consultancy. Both aim to help management, and both include analyses of circumstances, processes and opportunities. The audit, however, is essentially an evaluative process applying certain criteria that need to be agreed by all concerned before the audit takes place.

Data and information for audits

Reliable and relevant data are crucial in order to assess the quality of care. Many early audits looked solely at the standard of medical records and thus assessed the recording of information rather than the actual care of patients. This raises the question of what is meant by 'quality of care'. Is this to be measured by the input–output nexus, by the actual outcomes of care, by the process of care or by a combination of these?

'Care' is a potentially more complex concept than 'services'. Services relate to outputs, to the transformation of resources into identifiable – even tangible – items, operations, domiciliary help and physical aids for mobility being a few examples. Care has much more to do with *process* and *outcome*, with the nature of interaction between staff and prospective or actual patients and their families, and with the perceived benefits that result from intervention.

Data collected in order to inform people about the 'nature of interaction' (*process*) have to be qualitative and largely subjective. On the other hand, data gathered in order to assess the impact of health care interventions on intended beneficiaries can be both quantitative and qualitative.

Satisfaction surveys

These surveys are carried out mainly in a hospital setting, although there are instances in which primary health care clinics and community nursing services have also initiated surveys. Many hospitals have introduced complaints and suggestions channels for patients, and in this case, a member of the administrative staff will be designated to take on the responsibility for co-ordinating a response to patients' and families' views.

As a general observation, professionals have developed knowledge about what 'quality' means for them, but they have not focused on patients' views. Yet, where efforts have been made to invite lay persons to comment on their experience of the clinical process, the design and detail of, for example, patient questionnaires have often been seriously flawed. The defects have resulted from three main sources:

1. Survey questionnaires have been designed from a 'top-down' viewpoint by administrators/managers whose criteria of what are priority issues in the area of quality assurance – of what defines a high-quality service – may not be shared by users.
2. The questions are often limited in scope as a result of the particular perspective of management, and they tend to be 'closed' questions that do not permit respondents to select their own topics for comment.
3. The concern with specific aspects of the organisation's services and facilities – such as 'hotel' aspects, waiting times and physical amenities – ignores the fact that the total service package experienced by patients is multifaceted.

Furthermore, research into how patients reach decisions about their satisfaction levels indicates that the assumptions on which many surveys are based are suspect. The findings (Williams 1994) show that satisfaction:

- Is not related to the degree of difference between the benefits desired and those actually received
- May be a reflection of the role that patients adopt in relation to health professionals, for example accepting medical paternalism
- Is correlated with age: the older the person, the more likely there is to be a relatively high level of satisfaction
- Takes very little account of technical competence, which most patients take for granted, and has more to do with the behavioural aspects of the care process, such as adequate information and communication.

In devising patient satisfaction surveys, there may be a simplistic assumption that there is a strong link between 'satisfaction' and the 'fulfilment of expectations'. *Discrepancy theory* posits a gap between desires and what is experienced as a proportion of those desires. *Fulfilment theory* is based on the idea of a difference between the rewards desired and those fulfilled. *Equity theory* refers to an individual's perceived balance between inputs and outputs compared with those of other people. Yet the literature review carried out by Williams (1994) concluded that 'patients often do not evaluate in terms of being satisfied' and that 'we would expect that a wide range of behaviour to be [sic] permissible with only socially extreme behaviour causing dissatisfaction' (p. 514).

Much research still needs to be carried out in order to steer patient satisfaction surveys away from superficial data that have no convincing theoretical foundation. Williams' research highlights the need to take into consideration a number of variables that might exert an influence upon expressed degrees of satisfaction with health care services, for example individuals' knowledge and the prior experience of services. As previously stated, he notes that satisfaction may be a reflection of the *role* that patients adopt in relation to health professionals. Patients' apparent satisfaction with the services received could be an acceptance of medical paternalism rather than a true evaluation of the process of care. Finally, meta-research – research comparing research methods and resulting data – has indicated that quantitatively measured expressions of satisfaction derived from closed questions tend to be high while qualitative data as a response to open questions reveal greater levels of disquiet.

Furthermore, a random selection and analysis of existing and widely used patient satisfaction questionnaires underlines two reservations about this method of trying to assess the quality of health care experienced by patients. First, the questionnaire as a medium of expressing opinions is limited, particularly when it is constructed with exclusively or predominantly 'tick box' response options. Second, the use of questionnaires is possibly a popular means of trying to elicit people's opinions because they are relatively cost-effective to administer and analyse whereas the potentially more fruitful adoption of group interviews and more free-ranging discussions on a one-to-one level conducted at various stages of patient experience, for example, during hospital stay and at one or two periods after discharge, may prove unattractive to managers because they are relatively costly.

A careful look at the first six questions assembled from different patient satisfaction questionnaires demonstrates the deceptively instructive nature of this form of data collection.

Extracts from patient satisfaction surveys

(Patients are asked to tick boxes, for example 'Very satisfied', to 'Very dissatisfied', or 'Excellent' to 'Poor'.)

1. Were you satisfied with the way you were treated in the hospital?
2. How would you rate the meals you had during your stay?
3. Did the nursing care you received come up to your expectations?
4. Was your length of stay in the hospital too long, too short or about right?
5. Were the physical amenities of a high quality?
6. Did the clinical staff explain to you the type of treatment you were to receive?

Question 1, for example, uses the ambiguous word 'treated' and makes no allowance for an 'it depends' response, which would enable patients or ex-patients to discriminate between good 'treatment' relating to one aspect of their hospitalisation or to particular episodes compared with other aspects or episodes that did not amount to good 'treatment', although – as we have noted – how one patient interprets 'treated' may differ markedly from how another patient might understand the word.

Question 2 suffers from the same defect as question 1 in not affording an opportunity for respondents to distinguish between different meals. Breakfasts might have been uniformly, occasionally or never 'excellent' or 'good', whereas lunches could have rated as 'satisfactory' most of the time.

Question 3 assumes that patients entered hospital with expectations about the quality of nursing care.

Question 4 is surely seeking to discover people's perception of the acceptability of the length of stay rather than to offer a judgement on the clinical wisdom of the duration of their time in hospital.

One of the problems with question 5 is the lack of precision with respect to the term 'physical amenities': does it refer to the comfort of the beds, the condition and cleanliness of rooms, seating arrangements in waiting areas – or all or some of these?

Finally, question 6 does not explain what is meant by 'clinical staff'. If the term includes medical as well as nursing and para-medical staff, patients have no scope for expressing opinions about these sectors of the clinical staff, instead being forced into an aggregate evaluation that might register a severe distortion of their real feelings. If this type of ill-conceived question structure prompts a negative response, what information is it giving about what action should be taken and where?

In trying to cut corners, the architects of many patient satis-faction questionnaires exclude the logical device of using filter questions followed by an option to add an explanatory note, for example 'If you have answered "too short" to question 4 would you please explain why you gave this answer.' Another ques-tionnaire devised by an English university department consists of well over 100 questions – a potentially intolerable challenge to recuperating patients – but its central flaw lies in its attempt to cover all aspects of patient experience with a predetermined set of closed questions, the responses to which are likely to bear little resemblance to the person's actual experience. In short, flawed questions produce flawed data, which result in misinfor-mation, and misinformation should never be allowed to form the basis for decision-making. As Whitfield and Baker (1992) have commented:

Poor questionnaires act as a form of censorship imposed on patients. They give misleading results, limit the opportunity of patients to express their concerns about different aspects of care, and can encourage profes-sionals to believe that patients are satisfied when in fact they are highly discontented. (p. 152)

Consulting the public

Patient satisfaction surveys, complaints procedures, public meet-ings and citizens' forums are all methods of enabling people to contribute to health care planning decisions and policy develop-ment. Exhortations by governments to involve members of the public in health care planning can be interpreted as being consistent with a more participative orientation to policy-making in the public sector. While it could be applauded as a departure from the traditional democratic model of policy-making that assumes the right, once elected, of a government to create policies without direct reference to its populace, public participation can raise a number of issues. These centre on:

- The decision-making level at which participation plays a contributing role
- The extent to which such participation actually influences the decision-making process
- The degree to which the participants reflect and represent the wider public
- The potential conflict or incompatibility between lay and professional judgements
- The validity of public opinion, having regard to some of the means used in order to collect qualitative data.

Furthermore, while it might be politically 'correct' to talk and write about 'citizen empowerment', 'patients' charters' and 'public participation', little research has been carried out into the public's own views about becoming 'empowered' and 'included'. We might feel obligated, for example, to discredit or disprove the following hypotheses *before* embarking on a programme of lay involvement in health care planning decisions:

1. People expect professionals to make decisions.
2. The people can change the government through their vote – that is sufficient power.
3. Professionals would abdicate from their responsibility if they had to consult patients.
4. Ordinary people have neither the time nor the interest.
5. People might want to be more involved at the personal level but not at the strategic or operational levels of service planning and provision.
6. Participation raises people's expectations which might be difficult or impossible to satisfy.
7. It is difficult to define 'communities' so to talk about 'community empowerment' is not practicable.
8. To give no more power is more honest than to offer only token participation.

9. People might not act responsibly or in the general interest;
10. People with problems do not want to be burdened with the responsibility for decision-making.

Even if we could convincingly demolish each of the above objections to citizen participation in decision-making, there are methodological problems in gathering data. It has already been noted, in referring to the initiatives undertaken in one state in the USA and in one region of England, that there may be difficulties in ensuring that the sample used in the surveys is closely representative of the population at large. In patient satisfaction questionnaires, questions can be constructed that impose on respondents a very limited set of options. Raising such problems of data validity is not intended to undermine efforts to add the consumer perspective to health care planning, but it is meant as a cautionary observation that the methods of data collection should be selected in order to ensure that the results accurately reflect the views of participants.

One area of decision-making that would probably present a convincingly moral argument for lay involvement is planning treatment and care at the individual level, and there is an increasing focus on the contribution that patients can make towards assessing the impact of health care interventions. On a one-to-one level, it should not be difficult methodologically to provide a channel for the meaningful and accurate expression of individual opinions (Entwistle *et al*. 1998).

Methods of measuring health care outcomes

Any measure of outcome needs to be both longitudinal and multi-dimensional in order to capture the changing picture. (Kelly *et al*. 1994, p. 268)

Treatments that lead to successful removal of disease and yet do not improve quality of life or health status can be viewed as successful in only a limited technical and medical sense. (Jenkinson 1994)

It is clear from these two quotations that determining the 'success' of medical interventions may be more complex and problematic than merely relying upon clinicians' judgements of the efficacy of treatment. In the days before advanced techniques in medical practice and control over diseases through immunisation programmes, three outcome indicators were used; Florence Nightingale devised a simple classification of patient outcome following a period in hospital – on discharge, patients were classified as being either (a) relieved, (b) unrelieved, or (c) dead. This classification was used in some UK teaching hospitals until the late 1960s (Bate 1994).

In 1991, Bardsley and Cole set out a list of outcome indicators that included both clinically based measures and measures of the patients' perceptions of their own health:

1. Deaths and survival
2. Major adverse events after discharge, for example readmission to hospital
3. Treatment complications: problems after surgery, such as wound infection
4. Treatment success
5. Relief of individuals' symptoms or problems
6. Changes in general health status.

This composite set of measures is wholly consistent with a more holistic approach to health care interventions and their 'success' as perceived by professionals and patients.

One health profile includes, under the heading 'Subjective Health Status', pain, disability, anxiety, depression, social isolation, embarrassment and difficulties in carrying on daily life. Health care outcomes involve, according to these analyses, technical, psychological and social meaning as professionals and patients make sense, from their own perspectives of the impact of interventions on the service recipient.

One of the most influential schemes devised to assess the quality of health care was developed by Donabedian in the USA. He argued that, while the most direct route to an assessment of the quality of care is an examination of that care (the *process*), an assessment of what he designated *structure* and *outcome* allows another, indirect approach to measurement (Donabedian 1966).

While Donabedian's general approach is useful as a variation on the system model presented in Chapter 5, today's emphasis is more likely to be on attempting to measure *outcome* as a multi-faceted component of the health care experience. Donabedian recognised that, in the health care services, three factors were central to determining the 'quality' of care provided. These are:

- The *technical* dimension: the application skills and technology (competence of practitioners)
- The *interaction* between practitioner and client (the 'bedside manner')
- The *amenities and settings* within which the care or treatment takes place (for example the 'hotel facilities' in hospital).

These components were translated by Donabedian into his structure – process – outcome model of assessment in which 'structure' involves a set of inputs, including human and financial resources, facilities and the structure of the organisation, 'process' includes the giving and receiving of care, and 'outcome' refers to changes in health status and patient satisfaction. The important contribution that Donabedian made to the analysis of where resources could be most aptly and cost-effectively placed lies in his recognition of the patient's perspective as a crucial component in assessing the complex concept of quality of health care.

Impairment, disability and handicap

A clear example of the distinction between a clinical assessment of outcome and a personal interpretation can be found in the WHO's (1980) classification of impairments, disabilities and handicaps. The WHO recognised three different consequences of disease.

Impairments are defined as 'any loss or abnormality of psychological, physiological or anatomical structure or function'. Such phenomena are clinically diagnosed and defined. They are listed as:

- Intellectual impairments
- Other psychological impairments
- Language impairments
- Aural impairments
- Ocular impairments
- Visceral impairments
- Skeletal impairments
- Disfiguring impairments
- Generalised, sensory and other impairments.

Disabilities are the functional consequences of impairments. They indicate failures in accomplishment and are classified under nine headings:

- Behaviour disabilities
- Communication disabilities
- Personal care disabilities
- Locomotor disabilities
- Body disposition disabilities
- Dexterity disabilities
- Situational disabilities
- Particular skill disabilities
- Other activity restrictions.

Handicaps refer to the social consequences of impairments and disabilities. In essence, a handicap is a disadvantage experienced by an individual who suffers from an impairment or disability. These handicaps are listed below:

- Orientation handicap
- Physical independence handicap
- Mobility handicap
- Occupation handicap
- Social integration handicap
- Economic self-sufficiency handicap
- Other handicap.

There are some conceptual problems, however, with these classifications. The criterion by which *disabilities* and *handicaps* are defined rests upon an assessment of the individual's capacity to function in the manner or within the range considered normal for a human being. There might be room for dispute over what qualifies as 'normal' in this context. One instance of a handicap is a limitation on the ability to present a favourable image in social situations, another criterion that is open to different interpretations. Despite some reservations about classifying certain behaviour as that which might be expected of the average human being, there are advantages in recognising the potential *consequences* of impairments:

1. Additional dimensions are attached to the notion of 'health outcome'. A clinical evaluation of a particular treatment as

being 'successful' or 'efficacious' can predict only to a limited degree the extent to which an individual patient will suffer from a disability and, even less, from a handicap that is often socially determined.

2. The classifications, therefore, introduce the key component of personal experience – the patient's perspective – as being essential to a full assessment of any health care intervention.

3. They also underline the point that an *outcome* is not to be seen as a fixed 'end-state' but as an *ongoing* personal experience. In a sense, we could argue that this concept of a health care outcome recognises that the clinically successful operation, treatment or provision of a prosthetic device (for example an artificial limb) may not have a positive effect as judged by the criteria of disability or handicap.

Examples

> A clinically successful mastectomy might result in a disfiguring impairment, which, in turn, leads to a psychological impairment and a consequent problem with 'social integration'.
>
> Left-handed people who would not be diagnosed as suffering from any impairment are likely to experience mild forms of dexterity disability since it is less easy for them to accomplish a number of day-to-day tasks and functions: writing from left to right, using scissors and even shaking hands comes more naturally to right-handed people.
>
> Relatively poor eyesight may be improved by wearing spectacles and thus lead to none of the nine WHO disabilities, but this might debar that person from certain occupations that demand excellent vision.

Health care outcomes, according to this broader approach to evaluating 'success' or 'effectiveness', depend not only on the skills and competencies of practitioners, but also on the individual and on social attitudes. Townsend (1962) coined the term 'structured dependency' to describe the way in which a social system can impose a dependent relationship between certain citizens and the state. On a fairly superficial level, this is exemplified by the creation of a statutory age of retirement from paid employment, although exceptions are made in many countries, with the effect that some salaried professionals, such as

Members of Parliament and judges, are permitted to continue after the national age limit.

Other, more implicit policies operate that appear to devalue and exclude from the mainstream of society's activities people who are not physically or mentally 'normal'. In many countries, attempts to counter such inequities have been consolidated in antidiscrimination legislation seeking to enable persons with impairments to have equal access not only to buildings and public transport, but also to jobs and career opportunities that are taken for granted by non-impaired individuals.

QALYs, DALYs and Euroquol

Initiatives have been taken to combine data encompassing both clinical and lay assessments of health care outcome into a formula that can be applied in order to make more publicly defensible decisions about the prioritising of finite resources.

One notable attempt to combine such assessments is the QALY. Rosser and Kind (1978) asked various groups of doctors to describe the criteria by which they judged the severity of illness in their patients. From their responses, two key components of severity were identified: observed disability and subjective distress. From these components, and after structured interviews with 70 raters (medical patients, psychiatric patients, nurses, healthy volunteers and doctors), a two-dimensional classification of illness states was developed ranging from 'No disability' to 'Unconscious' and from 'No distress' to 'Severe distress'. This scale was further developed by Rosser, taking into account additional, subjectively experienced attributes of the after-effects of treatment. Median values of the final scores were transformed so that a score of zero was attributed to death, and perfect health with no distress was scored at 1. Negative values refer to conditions that are regarded as being worse than death.

The formula for devising QALYs was adopted as the foundation for the Oregon plan described in Chapter 6. Despite its shortcomings, it does recognise and acknowledge that, in making decisions about where it is most cost-effective to assign resources, two key elements have to be part of the equation:

1. The patient's own assessment of his or her physical, mental and social state

2. The medical prognosis of the probable effects of treatments and care in terms of the duration and quality of benefits to the patient.

Table 9.1   Transformed quality of life values

Disability	Distress			
	A	**B**	**C**	**D**
1	1.000	0.995	0.990	0.967
2	0.990	0.986	0.973	0.932
3	0.980	0.972	0.956	0.942
4	0.964	0.956	0.942	0.870
5	0.946	0.935	0.900	0.700
6	0.875	0.845	0.680	0.000
7	0.677	0.564	0.000	−1.486
8	−1.028			

The disability adjusted life-year (DALY) is a variant of the QALY, and the Euroquol was devised in order to simplify the method of compiling a list of different health states. Whereas QALYs were identified through a series of interviews with health care practitioners and lay people, the Euroquol used postal questionnaires to construct a framework for analysis (Jenkinson 1994).

Evidence-based practice

One criticism of the QALY approach to health care decision-making is the fallibility of the medical profession in forecasting, with any degree of accuracy, the probable impact of their treatment on a patient's health and general well-being. Cochrane (1972) was an early exponent of a much more rigorous methodology in order to test the efficacy of clinical interventions. He promoted the need for randomised control trials, in which experimental and control groups are used so that the key variable – treatment of some kind – can be isolated and checked for its effect.

Although the principles expounded by Cochrane have gained general acceptance, the inherent ethical and methodological

problems involved have led to alternative, or at least complementary, approaches to establishing valid data on which planning decisions can be founded. Some of these are:

- *Observation studies:* compare professional A using procedure
  'a' with professional B using procedure 'b'
- *Before-and-after studies:* compare professional B who changes
  from 'a' to 'b' with professional A who adheres to 'a' throughout
- *Pragmatic trials:* whereas randomised controlled trials seek to
  draw conclusions about scientific hypotheses, pragmatic trials
  try to produce evidence about the relative merits of different
  procedures or technologies in normal practice
- *Testable assertions:* the refinement of assumptive statements to
  a form that is precise, one-dimensional and, therefore,
  amenable to testing in terms of its efficacy.

The quest for harder evidence about which treatments 'work'
has proved to be provocative. It has gained support from health
care managers in the UK, concerned as they are with the most
cost-effective use of resources and with PIs that can be used to
make comparisons between hospitals' clinical 'success rates'. It
has also attracted positive and negative responses from medical
practitioners. On the positive side, Roberts *et al.* (1996) refute the
conventional wisdom that asserts a mismatch between infinite
demand and finite resources in the health care arena. They argue
that huge amounts of money are allocated to treatments that have
no hard evidential basis for their application. What they advocate
is the development of assertions or hypotheses that lend themselves to being tested for their efficacy. In this way, resources can
be allocated to health care interventions of *proven* efficacy.

The results of tried-and-tested treatments can then be communicated to other medical colleagues in order to influence clinical
practice. According to Appleby *et al.* (1995), evidence-based
medicine can encourage a more considered approach to management, priority-setting and policy-making. It is concerned with
answering the questions, Does it work? and, Is it worth it?

Views contrary to those of the evidence-based medicine
'movement' have been articulated, for example by Fowler (1997),
who dismisses this approach as something of a slur upon the
professional judgement of the medical profession and as a built-
in method for rejecting or delaying medical advances.

Summary

Logic dictates that, in any enterprise involving the spending of tax-payers' money, decisions about where the money should be spent ought to be based on evidence in the form of carefully constructed data. Health care professionals are primarily accountable to each individual patient, although they are becoming more and more accountable to management in many settings where efficiency and cost-effectiveness co-exist alongside the criteria of medical efficacy and general quality of care.

In many societies, hospital authorities and primary and secondary care organisations are also directly accountable to the government. Whereas, in the past, the autonomy of doctors to apply their knowledge and expertise was unquestioned, the influence of health economists as policy advisers to politicians has served to emphasise the obligation to 'prove the case' for investing resources in this area of health care rather than that, in this form of treatment rather than another.

The 'proof', however, is not to be found exclusively in clinical judgements. Decision-makers who are central to the planning process are looking more and more to a blend of highly quantitative data and the much more personal, experiential data provided by the other experts, namely those people who have been the recipients of health care interventions.

Items for discussion

1. Construct counterarguments to the list of 10 items presented in this chapter that argue against involving members of the public and patients in contributing to health care planning decisions.
2. Apart from questionnaires, what alternative or additional data collection methods could be used in order to discover patients' opinions about the health care services they have experienced?

Chapter 10 Health care planning: current and future issues

Decisions about the size of budgets to be allocated from government resources to health care services and the prioritising of the budget according to perceived needs and demands are continually exercising the minds of politicians and their advisers. Despite criticisms of the planning process, the need to respond to change in a systematic and scheduled manner will remain a central concern of governments and health care organisations. How to respond is also an important matter. If health care systems are to plan for the resourcing of services, there need to be methods for anticipating the potential impact of developing and, possibly, innovative forms of intervention. Planners – now more than ever before – will have to be proactive rather than reactive, such is the potential pace of change in many countries.

Products and processes

Davey and Popay (1993) make a distinction between (1) invention and innovation; and (2) product and process innovations. They describe 'invention' as referring to the generation of new knowledge from fundamental scientific research and 'innovation' as the application of inventions and new scientific insights to produce goods and services, that is, the *development* part of research and development. They also make the point, to be discussed later, that it is usually easier to introduce innovative products than it is to implement innovative processes.

Prompting the design of many innovations is medical technology. This term has been comprehensively defined as:

The drugs, devices and medical and surgical procedures used in medical care and the organisation and supportive systems within which such care is provided. (US Office of Technology Assessment, quoted in Davey and Popay 1993).

This definition includes both product and process forms of technology, which are often intimately related. One technological change may lead to another. For example, the development of new anaesthetics (a product innovation) has enabled patients to recover sufficiently quickly to be discharged within a few hours of surgery. This has had the effect of increasing the use of day surgery (a process innovation) in order to minimise the cost of hospital care. In turn, the spread of day surgery is encouraging surgeons to develop new, less invasive procedures, enabling new types of operation to be undertaken as day cases.

Variations in the extent to which innovations are applied in different countries may be attributable to a number of factors other than the relative wealth of those countries. Political, religious, cultural, social and legal considerations may have an influence. Organ transplants and the consumption of pharmaceuticals, for example, pose religious, cultural and economic questions. Resources made available for the adoption of new technologies may also be affected by the structure and organisation of different health care systems. In situations where central government exerts a high degree of control over the total level of spending on health care, the funding of applied technology may be accorded a different priority compared with policies in those countries where health care is funded predominantly through insurance schemes.

Planning in a hospital setting

The introduction of new technology into a hospital setting will depend, to a large extent, on the perceived benefits set against costs. In addition, hospital managers and administrators will have to take into account the possible 'shelf-life' of new product technologies. New scanning techniques, such as magnetic resonance imaging, have to be financed on a long-term basis. Technological products of this kind have to be updated and upgraded, in terms of both hardware and software. Planners, therefore, have to forecast recurring as well as capital costs.

Introducing process innovations can prove to be difficult even though the change may not adversely affect running costs or might even reduce them. Stocking (1984) examined the reasons why a number of hospitals in a specified area of the UK refused to implement new recommendations made by a Royal Commission. The most commonly expressed complaint by patients, which led to the recommendations, was the early waking time. Despite the efforts of hospital administrators, nursing staff resisted any change because they claimed that there were insufficient night staff to manage the process of allowing patients to stay up later. Therefore, they put patients to bed earlier and were justified in waking them up at an early hour.

Future developments

Since the acquisition and allocation of resources lies at the heart of health care planning, much more innovative ways in which to manage these resources will need to be discovered and applied. Not least, of course, is the complex question of the priority given to public health expenditure in the sphere of health promotion and illness prevention compared with the emphasis and consequent funding assigned to health care interventions. Care in hospitals is relatively expensive. Can ways be found, as a result of more product innovations, to deliver health care services to patients in their own homes?

The opposition by clinical personnel to maternity confinement at home has been justified by stressing the need for scrupulous standards of hygiene. The move in many societies to reduce the length of stay in hospital for non-complicated births bears witness to policy and planning in action. Occupying a hospital bed for 24 or 48 hours rather than for 72 hours or more obviously saves money. Could further savings be made by admitting to hospital only those cases in which there was a clear medical need to do so?

A policy move to focus care in the community rather than institutional settings also stimulates debate about the potential for 'rationalising' health and social care resources. When does *medical care* become *personal tending*? Do people in need of support require a community nurse or a skilled home help? To what extent do health and social care workers duplicate each others' services? Over the whole health care field, how can the skills of various medical, nursing and paramedical staff be used to best advantage so that tasks are assigned to the most appropriately cost-effective level?

One recent process innovation proposed in Britain is the one-stop high street health shop linked to a computer screen, where GP and patient can discuss diagnosis and the latest treatment options. Hospital appointments, if appropriate, will be booked while the patient waits, and hospital test results will be despatched electronically to the doctor's screen, prescriptions being similarly despatched to the pharmacy. Each patient will have a lifelong electronic record available 24 hours a day online to doctors or via a laptop to paramedics at the scene of an accident. Telemedicine will play an increasingly significant role in the diagnosis and treatment of patients (Murray 1999).

Advances in medical technology will, however, continue to create as well as solve problems. The availability of high-tech treatments such as laser applications, genetic probes to help to identify defective genes, and fertility treatments tend to raise public expectations and fuel demand. The success of health care systems can be gauged by the extent to which policy-makers and planners are able to contain expenditure and, at the same time, maintain public confidence and support.

Summary

In this and the preceding chapters, some of the key concepts used in the analysis of health care policy and planning have been identified and discussed. Since this is an introductory text, references are made to further reading, which will, of course, need to be updated as new published material is produced. The main, integrating message that is presented here is that frameworks to aid thinking about health care policy and planning are intended as useful devices in order to help to clarify current and future debates about how best to develop high-quality health care systems; additionally, such systems will reflect the particular social, political and cultural contexts in which they are located.

Good health is a universal aspiration; the means of achieving this nationally and globally will be a continuing and complex challenge.

Key Concepts in Health Care Policy and Planning

Items for discussion

1. Consider the different priorities that might be accorded to aspects of health promotion, primary care and hospital care in developed and less-developed countries.
2. In what ways are current and potential developments in medical technology and research likely to reduce or increase demand for certain health care services?

References

* Denotes core texts recommended for further reading.

Alford, R (1975) *Health Care Politics.* Chicago: University of Chicago Press

Althusser, L (1971) *Lenin and Philosophy and Other Essays.* London: New Left Books

Appleby, J, Walshe, K and Ham, C (1995) *Acting on the Evidence.* NAHAT Research Paper. Birmingham: National Association of Health Authorities and Trusts (NAHAT)

Arnstein, L (1969) 'A ladder of citizen participation in the USA'. *Journal of the American Institute of Planners* 35(4)

Atkinson, R and Moon, G (1994) *Urban Policy in Britain.* London: Macmillan

Baggott, R (1998) *Health and Health Care in Britain.* London: Macmillan

Bardsley, M and Cole, J (1991) 'Measured steps to outcome'. *Health Service Journal,* 17 October: 18–20

Bartholomew, J (1994) 'Laws that backfire'. *The Times,* 17 December, p. 12

Bate, L (1994) 'Information for assessment of health outcomes'. *Health Management Update* February 1–3

Bowie, C, Richardson, A and Sykes, W (1995) 'Consulting the public about health service priorities'. *British Medical Journal* **311**: 1155–8

Bradshaw, J (1972) 'A taxonomy of human need', in McLachlan, G (ed.) *Problems and Progress in Medical Care: Essays in Current Research.* Oxford: Oxford University Press

Braye, S and Preston-Shoot, M (1995) *Empowering Practice in Social Care.* Buckingham: Open University Press

Buttery, Y (1994) *Evaluating Medical Audit.* London: Clinical Accountability Service Planning and Evaluation (CASPE)

Campling, EA, Lunn, JA and Devlin, HB (1990) *The Report of the National Enquiry into Peri-operative Deaths.* NCEPOD

Challis, L, Klein, R and Webb, A (1988) *Joint Approaches to Social Policy.* Cambridge: Cambridge University Press

*Coast J, Donovan, J and Frankel, S (eds) (1996) *Priority Setting: The Health Care Debate.* London: John Wiley & Sons

Cochrane, A (1972) *Effectiveness and Efficiency: Random Reflections on Health Services.* London: Nuffield Provincial Hospitals Trust

Cronbach, LJ (1963) 'Course improvement through evaluation'. *Teachers College Record* **64**: 672–83

Cronbach, LJ (1982) *Designing Evaluations of Education and Social Programs.* San Francisco: Jossey-Bass

References

Davey, B and Popay, J (eds) (1993) *Dilemmas in Health Care*. Buckingham: Open University Press

Deakin, N (1987) *The Politics of Welfare*. London: Methuen

Department of the Environment (1992) *Policy Evaluation: The Role of Social Research*. London: HMSO

Department of Health (1989) *Working for Patients*. London: HMSO

Department of Health (1998) *Our Healthier Nation*. London: HMSO

Department of Health and Social Security (1976) *Priorities for Health and Social Services in England*. London: HMSO

Department of Health and Social Security (1980) *Inequalities in Health* (the Black Report). London: HMSO

Department of Health and Social Security (1992) *The Health of the Nation*. London: HMSO

Donabedian, A (1966) 'Evaluating quality of medical care'. *Millbank Memorial Fund Quarterly* **44**: 169

Doyal, L and Gough, I (1979) *A Theory of Human Need*. London: Macmillan

Dror, Y (1989) *Design of Policy Sciences*. New York: Elsevier

Durkheim, E (1938) *The Rules of Sociological Method*. New York: Free Press

Easton, D (1965) *Framework for Political Analysis*. Englewood Cliffs, NJ: Prentice Hall

Elmore, RF (1978) 'Organizational models of social program implementation'. *Public Policy*, **26**(2): 185–228

Entwistle, V, Sowden, AJ and Watt, IS (1998) 'Evaluating interventions to promote patient involvement in decision-making: by what criteria should effectiveness be judged?' *Journal of Health Service Research Policy* **3**(2): 100–7

Etzioni, A (1967) Mixed scanning: a "third" approach to decision-making'. *Public Administration Review* **27**: 385–92

Field, MG (ed.) (1989) *Success and Crisis in National Health Systems*. London: Routledge

Flynn, R, Williams, G and Pickard, S (1996) *Markets and Networks: Contracting in Community Health Services*. Buckingham: Open University Press

Foucault, M (1973) *The Birth of the Clinic*. London: Tavistock

Fowler, PBS (1997) 'Evidence-based everything'. *Journal of Evaluation in Clinical Practice* **3**(3): 239–43

Freund, P and McGuire, M (1991) *Health, Illness and the Social Body*. Englewood Cliffs, NJ: Prentice Hall

Glynn, J, Perkins, DA and Stewart, S (1996) *Achieving Value for Money*. London: WB Saunders

Goffman, I (1968) *Asylum*. Harmondsworth: Penguin

Gramsci, A (1971) *Selections from Prison Notebooks*. London: Lawrence & Wishart

Granovetter, M (1985) 'Economic action and social structure: the problem of embeddedness'. *American Journal of Sociology* **91**(3): 481–510

Gray, C (1994) *Government Beyond the Centre*. London: Macmillan

Green, A (1995) 'The state of health planning in the '90s'. *Health Policy and Planning* **10**(1): 22–8

Gunn, L (1978) 'Why is implementation so difficult?' *Management Services in Government* **33**: 169–76

Hackman, R and Oldham, G (1980) *Work Redesign.* Reading, MA: Addison-Wesley

Ham, C (1981) *Policy making in the NHS.* London: Macmillan

Hamilton, J, Jenkins, D, King, C, MacDonald, B and Paulett, M (eds) (1977) *Beyond the Numbers Game: A Register in Educational Evaluation.* London: Macmillan

Harrison, S and Pollitt, C (1994) *Controlling Health Professionals.* Buckingham: Open University Press

Harrison, S, Hunter, DJ and Pollitt, C (1990) *The Dynamics of British Health Policy.* London: Unwin Hyman

Harrison, S, Hunter, DJ, Marnoch, G and Pollitt, C (1992) *Just Managing; Power and Culture in the NHS.* London: Macmillan

Hogwood, B and Gunn, L (1984) *Policy Analysis for the Real World.* Oxford: Oxford University Press

Holland, J and Blackburn, J (1998) *Whose Voice? Participatory Research and Policy Change.* London: Intermediate Technology Publications

Hood, CC (1976) *The Limits of Administration.* London: John Wiley & Sons

Hopkins, A (1991) 'Approaches to medical audit'. *Journal of Epidemiology and Community Health* **45**: 1–3

Hunter, D (1993) 'Care in the community: rhetoric or reality?' in Davey, B and Popay, J (eds) *Dilemmas in Health Care.* Buckingham: Open University Press

Illich, I (1975) *Limits to Medicine.* Harmondsworth: Penguin

*Jenkinson, C (ed.) (1994) *Measuring Health and Medical Outcomes.* London: University College Publishing

Kelly, M, Anderson, JR, Carey, LM and West, PB (1994) 'Some considerations for identifying quality measures of surgical outcome'. *Health Services Management Research* **7**(4): 265–70

Lee, K and Mills, D (1985) *Policy making and Planning in the Health Sector.* London: Croom Helm

Le Grand, J and Robinson, R (eds) (1994) *Evaluating the NHS Reforms.* London: King's Fund

Lewis, J and Glennerster, H (1996) *Implementing the New Community Care.* Buckingham: Open University Press

Lindblom, C (1959) 'The science of "muddling through"'. *Public Administration Review* **19**(3): 517–26

Lipsky, M (1980) *Street Level Bureaucracy.* New York: Russell Sage Foundation

Lukes, S (1974) *Power: A Radical View.* London: Macmillan

McKillip, J (1987) *Need Analysis: Tools for the Human Services and Education.* London: Sage

Marinker, M (ed.) (1994) *Controversies in Health Care Policies.* London: BMJ Publishing Group

References

Mark, A and Brennan, R (1995) 'De-marketing: managing demand in the UK National Health Service' *Public Money and Management* July–September: 17–22

Marx, K (1867) *Das Kapital* (1967 edition). London: Lawrence & Wishart

Maslow, A (1970) *Motivation and Personality.* New York: Harper & Row

Mathison, S (1992) 'An evaluation model for in-service teacher education'. *Evaluation and Program Planning* **15**: 255–61

Maxwell, R (1984) 'Quality assessment in health care'. *British Medical Journal* **288**: 166–203

Maynard, A (1991) 'Case for auditing audit'. *Health Service Journal* 18 July: 26

Mead, GH (1934) *Mind, Self and Society.* Chicago: University of Chicago Press

Miles, A (1988) *Women and Mental Illness: The Social Context of Female Neurosis.* Brighton: Wheatsheaf

Murray, I (1999) 'Hi-tech cures prescribed for health service'. *The Times,* 30 January: 18

Navarro, V (1978) *Class Struggle, the State and Medicine.* Oxford, Martin Robertson

Neuberger, J (1994) 'Availability of information in an open society', in Marinker, M (ed.) *Controversies in Health Care Policies.* London: BMJ Publishing Group

Oliver, M (1997) 'The disability movement is a new social movement'. *Community Development Journal* **32**(3): 244–51

Ovretveit, J, Mathias, P and Thompson, T (1997) *Interprofessional Working for Health and Social Care.* London: Macmillan

Palfrey, C, Phillips, C, Thomas, P and Edwards, D (1992) *Policy Evaluation in the Public Sector.* Aldershot: Avebury

Parsons, T (1967) *Sociological Theory and Modern Society.* New York: Glencoe Press

*Parsons, W (1995) *Public Policy: An Introduction to the Theory and Practice of Policy Analysis.* London: Edward Elgar

Patton, CV and Sawicki, DS (1986) *Basic Methods of Policy Analysis and Planning.* Englewood Cliffs, NJ: Prentice-Hall

*Phillips C, Palfrey, C and Thomas, P (1994) *Evaluating Health and Social Care.* London: Macmillan

Pressman, J and Wildavsky, A (1973) *Implementation.* Berkeley, CA: University of California Press

Ranson, S and Stewart, J (1994) *Management for the Public Domain.* London: Macmillan

Roberts, C, Lewis, P, Crosby, D, Dunn R and Grundy, P (1996) 'Prove it'. *Health Service Journal* March: 32–3

Roberts, H (ed.) (1992) *Women's Health Matters.* London: Routledge

Robinson, R (1993a) 'Economic evaluation and health care: what does it mean?' *British Medical Journal* **307**: 670–3

Robinson, R (1993b) 'Economic evaluation and health care: costs and cost-minimisation analysis'. *British Medical Journal* **307**: 726–8

Robinson, R (1993c) 'Economic evaluation and health care: cost-utility analysis'. *British Medical Journal* **307**: 859–62

Robinson, R (1993d) 'Economic evaluation and health care: the policy context'. *British Medical Journal* **307**: 994–6

Rosser, R and Kind, P (1978) 'A scale of valuations of states of illness: is there a social consensus?' *International Journal of Epidemiology* **7**(4): 346–58

Saville, J (1983) 'The origins of the welfare state', in Loney, M, Boswell, D and Clarke, J (eds) *Social Policy and Social Welfare*. Buckingham: Open University Press

Servian, R (1996) *Theorising Empowerment: Individual Power and Community Care*. University of Bristol: Policy Press

Simon, H (1957) *Administrative Behaviour*. New York: Free Press

Singapore Ministry of Health (1993) *Affordable Health Care*. Singapore: SNP Publishers

Smith, G and Cantley, C (1985) *Assessing Health Care: A Study in Organisational Evaluation*. Buckingham: Open University Press

Stocking, B (1984) *Initiative and Inertia: Case Studies in the NHS*. London: Nuffield Provincial Hospitals Trust

Thomas, P and Palfrey, C (1996) 'Evaluation: stakeholder-focused criteria'. *Social Policy and Administration* **30**(2): 125–42

Townsend, P (1962) *The Last Refuge*. London: Routledge & Kegan Paul

Tudor-Hart, J (1971) 'The inverse care law'. *Lancet* 27 February: 405–12

Vickers, G (1965) *The Art of Judgement*. London: Chapman & Hall

*Walt, G (1994) *Health Policy: An Introduction to Process and Power*. London: Zed Books

Weber, M (1948) 'Bureaucracy' in Gerth, C and Mills, CW (eds) *From Max Weber: Essays in Sociology*. New York: Oxford University Press

Welsh Health Planning Forum (1992) *Health and Social Care 2010: A Framework for Services*. Cardiff: Welsh Health Planning Forum

Wertz, RW and Wertz, DC (1979) *Lying-in: A History of Childbirth in America*. New York: Schocken

Whitfield, M and Baker, R (1992) 'Measuring patient satisfaction for audit in general practice'. *Quality Health Care* **3**: 151–8

Williams, B (1994) 'Patient satisfaction: a valid concept?' *Social Science and Medicine* **38**(4): 309–16

World Health Organisation (1946) *Constitution: Basic Documents*. Geneva: WHO

World Health Organisation (1978) *Report of the International Conference on Primary Health Care: Alma Ata 1977*. Geneva: WHO

World Health Organisation (1980) *International Classification of Impairments, Disabilities and Handicaps*. Geneva: WHO

World Health Organisation (1985) *Health for All by the Year 2000*. Geneva: WHO

Zola, K (1975) 'Medicine as an instrument of social control', in Cox, G and Mead, A (eds) *A Sociology of Medical Practice*. London: Collier-Macmillan

Index

A
aetiology 97
arithmetic mean 105
Arnstein's ladder 27–9
audit
  clinical 111
  cycle 111
  management 111, 112
  medical 112
Audit Commission 26

B
before-and-after studies 126
Belgium 7
Black Report 55
British Medical Association 20

C
capitalism 20, 86
capitalist societies 89
care in the community 4, 11, 40, 41, 53,
  55, 61, 69, 87, 130
choice(s) 12, 25, 28, 29, 53, 57, 61, 62,
  69, 72, 73, 92, 99
citizens' forums 117
civil servants/administrators 18, 31,
  32, 72, 97
codes of practice 110
competing rationalities 33, 99
complaints procedures 117
concepts 14, 39, 131
Conservative government 20
consumer(ism) 14, 22, 23, 29, 54, 91,
  110
  exit 24
  government as voice 244
co-operation 74
corporate planning 37, 75
cost–benefit analysis 37, 82
costs 58, 59, 61, 129
  health care 71, 103

opportunity 59, 87
outcome measures and 102
per treatment 77
Creutzfeldt-Jacob disease 98
cultural milieus 39
cultural pluralism 25

D
DALYs 124
data 95–127
  accessible 112
  analysed 95
  categorised 95
  comparative 109
  demographic 103
  epidemiological 99, 101, 103
  experiential 127
  hard 95, 106
  health care outcomes 99
  interpreted 95
  qualitative 111, 113, 115, 118
  quantitative 96, 109, 111, 113, 115,
    127
  soft 95, 101
  valid 126
decentralisation 90
decision-makers 98, 99
decision-making 9, 93, 98, 119
  improve 75
  operational 21, 24
  participatory approaches 25, 53
  the political process 117
  practitioner 21, 24
  process 31
  public involvement 10, 79
  rational models 9
  strategic 21, 24, 90
  system management approach 38
demand(s) 4, 48–9, 71, 73, 76, 82, 93–4,
  103, 126, 128
  de-marketing 71

Index

Index